Careers Beyond
Clinical Medicine

Careers Beyond Clinical Medicine

HEIDI MOAWAD, MD

OXFORD
UNIVERSITY PRESS

OXFORD
UNIVERSITY PRESS

Oxford University Press is a department of the University of Oxford.
It furthers the University's objective of excellence in research, scholarship,
and education by publishing worldwide.

Oxford   New York

Auckland   Cape Town   Dar es Salaam   Hong Kong   Karachi
Kuala Lumpur   Madrid   Melbourne   Mexico City   Nairobi
New Delhi   Shanghai   Taipei   Toronto

With offices in

Argentina   Austria   Brazil   Chile   Czech   Republic   France   Greece
Guatemala   Hungary   Italy   Japan   Poland   Portugal   Singapore
South Korea   Switzerland   Thailand   Turkey   Ukraine   Vietnam

Oxford is a registered trade mark of Oxford University Press in the UK and certain other countries.

Published in the United States of America by
Oxford University Press
198 Madison Avenue, New York, NY 10016

© Oxford University Press 2013

Library of Congress Cataloging-in-Publication Data

Moawad, Heidi.
Careers beyond clinical medicine / Heidi Moawad.
p. cm.
Includes bibliographical references and index.
ISBN 978-0-19-986045-6 (pbk.)
1. Medicine—Vocational guidance.   2. Career changes—Decision making.   I. Title.
R690.M63 2013
610.23—dc23
2012022310

The science of medicine is a rapidly changing field. As new research and clinical experience broaden
our knowledge, changes in treatment and drug therapy occur. The author and publisher of this work
have checked with sources believed to be reliable in their efforts to provide information that is accurate
and complete, and in accordance with the standards accepted at the time of publication. However, in
light of the possibility of human error or changes in the practice of medicine, neither the author, nor
the publisher, nor any other party who has been involved in the preparation or publication of this work
warrants that the information contained herein is in every respect accurate or complete. Readers are
encouraged to confirm the information contained herein with other reliable sources, and are strongly
advised to check the product information sheet provided by the pharmaceutical company for
each drug they plan to administer.

1 3 5 7 9 8 6 4 2
Printed in the United States of America
on acid-free paper

ACKNOWLEDGMENTS

I would like to thank all of the people who helped me with this project. The caring doctors who spent countless hours sharing their stories with me and telling me what they sincerely felt would be helpful for other physicians continue to use their talents to make the world a better place as they encourage others to do the same.

I appreciate the encouragement that Gail Weiss gave me when I first asked her what she thought of a book for physicians who are interested in pursuing non-traditional careers. Melissa Showers, always an amazing person who truly works hard to get things done, pointed me in the right direction. My friend and advisor Judy Edelstein, MD, has been a great support as I was formulating my ideas.

Craig Panner at Oxford University Press was such a wonderful advisor in helping me solidify my plan and guiding me in the new world of writing a book. My editor, Kathryn Winder, has been absolutely wonderful to work with. Thank you, Kathryn, for your constant genuine direction and advice.

And I would like to thank my husband, John, who has been so encouraging and loving throughout this process. Thank you for always being there to listen to my ideas and for being my partner and support in everything I do. I also want to thank my kids, Tommy, Lily, and Anna, for being so patient while I was busy working on this book.

CONTENTS

INTRODUCTION

As a physician, I have had the opportunity to work in several different capacities within the realm of medicine. I came from a medical community and, over the years, I have had an extended network of friends who are physicians. Early in my career I was drawn to the field of neurology and I truly loved treating patients. But I also craved insight into understanding who really pulls the strings in medicine and I wanted to grasp more about how healthcare works as a whole. As a clinical neurologist, my curiosity about what goes on behind the scenes in utilization review led to a conversation with a physician reviewer who was evaluating one of my diagnostic imaging requests. This friendly discussion opened the door to a remarkably pleasant and enlightening job at a leading healthcare management company.

I enjoyed my new work and appreciated the refreshing opportunity to see medicine from a different angle. I also felt gratified to have a voice and to be able to make a conscientious contribution to utilization review, an area that had previously made me feel powerless as a physician. Several years later, I took another angle professionally, as I started teaching human anatomy and physiology at the undergraduate level. I was drawn to teaching for several reasons. It provided me with the opportunity to provide a structure for students for a whole semester at a time, arranging a curriculum that ties the many features of human health together. It has also allowed me to introduce young people to the concept of effectively thinking about health issues from a scientific perspective.

I was caught by complete surprise, however, when many physicians, friends, friends of friends, former colleagues, and former classmates approached me to ask for advice on how to branch out into other areas of medicine, as I had. Initially, I encouraged people to use the same approaches that I had used in finding jobs. But then, over time, I realized that, while my experience was a very positive one, doctors who are looking for nonclinical careers may share some common threads, but do not fit into a one-size-fits-all mold.

As I listened to earnest stories of MDs searching for alternatives and direction, I learned that while my own initial motivation for exploring a nontraditional opportunity was an interest in learning about how other aspects of healthcare work, this is not the case for every doctor. I initially maintained a clinical neurology practice while working as a peer reviewer, and I also began to appreciate that this hybrid does not suit all physicians. In particular, my openness about my nonclinical pursuit was unusual. Most doctors who asked me about how to get into non-patient-care work did so quietly, and I became more aware of, and sensitive to, the stigma and professional and financial uncertainty associated with leaving clinical medicine.

Despite the significant demand, there remains very little reliable information regarding nonclinical jobs and opportunities for physicians. Straightforward facts about salaries, job availability, job security, and the right approach to finding nonclinical medical work are scant and vague. Most doctors simply do not know whom to ask about these issues. Furthermore, there is no training program or formal route for physicians who are interested in exploring opportunities outside of conventional medical practice. There are no guidelines for doctors who want to combine clinical work with alternative work, and no clear strategies for transitional plans.

To help fill this void, I began speaking to doctors who have achieved satisfaction and success in a broad range of nonclinical medical careers. I found many physicians who have pursued exciting and challenging paths and whose stories offered a wide expanse of direction for fellow physicians. These physicians have graciously shared their personal experiences, their advice, and their valuable insight, so that they may help other doctors effectively approach this decision and career modification. Doctors have a lot to say concerning why they contemplated doing something with their careers besides the conventional practice of medicine and how they achieved their alternative goals.

Many of the MDs who contributed their stories for this book explained that there was no set of instructions for them when they paved their own ways. Sometimes they found their nontraditional jobs without a great deal of support or encouragement. As a result, a repeated theme that I have been hearing is, "This is what I wish someone told me."

Doctors who regularly evaluate and hire physician candidates in several nonclinical areas describe which qualities they look for in a job applicant. Recruiters have provided candid information about salaries, job availability, and physician career trends. This book connects the many physicians who want honest direction about nonclinical opportunities, with a wide variety of experts who have the elusive, unfiltered, behind-the-scenes facts.

The result is a resource for doctors, which contains valuable information that can be used when considering whether to pursue a nonclinical route and how to achieve professional objectives. The first section examines the factors involved in the often difficult and complicated decision to leave clinical medicine, and provides a balanced approach to deciding what to do next. The second section describes the many opportunities that are available for doctors along with their important numbers: job availability, salaries, work hours, expectations, and work environment. The third section provides detailed instructions and guidelines for effectively attaining and succeeding at the career path that is right for you along with real-life success stories.

I hope that as you read about the reasons that other doctors have expressed for seeking alternatives you gain validation of your feelings about your role in medicine and form an honest evaluation of what you want to do next. You can find answers to the many questions about available opportunities for doctors that you do not know whom to ask. And you will be able to use the tools necessary to evaluate suitable ways for you to use your education, experience, and skills with consideration for your professional and personal needs as you make this decision. You can weigh objective facts about productive, well-respected nonclinical opportunities, and find a realistic roadmap to achieving professional satisfaction to achieve your professional goals. You will always be a doctor—and that is a great thing. As you decide how to approach the next chapter of your professional life, you can be assured that the advanced qualifications, skills, and experiences that you gained as a physician will be of great benefit to you and to others as you remain a doctor beyond clinical medicine. Most of the doctors who contributed their advice for this book have given me permission to use their names. A few of the physicians who generously shared their insights and stories have requested privacy, and therefore their names have been changed, while their valuable advice remains available for you.

SECTION ONE

SHOULD I STAY OR SHOULD I GO?

1

If I'm a Good Doctor, Why Do I Want to Do Something Else?

Like many physicians, you may have considered the idea of looking for another career, profession, or endeavor that does not directly follow the traditional definition of being a doctor. Many doctors have effectively redefined their careers beyond clinical practice at various points between the early days of medical school to even some time after retirement.

The doctors who have embarked on nonclinical careers are as diverse in their personalities as can be and cannot be confined to any typical stereotype. For physicians, the decision to explore nontraditional work arises at different professional levels and with varied financial stability. There is a wide scope of physician personalities who embark on alternative career routes, including business-oriented MDs, innovative doctors, intense physicians, relaxed physicians, those who follow altruistic passions, social personalities, Democrats, Republicans, conservatives, religious individuals, hippies, and artistic physicians. I have even known physicians living outside the United States who have decided to take their careers in other directions. Nevertheless, their stories reflect that what these doctors have in common is that they are good doctors who are hard working and well respected professionally.

One thing that everyone agrees on is that it is normal to experience conflicted feelings about whether to stay in clinical medicine or to leave. So it is critical to thoroughly address any and all facets of uncertainty early on in the process to clarify for yourself exactly *why* you want to turn the page to the next chapter in your career. Your incentives for leaving clinical practice or trying something new play a considerable role in determining what you choose to do next and have a substantial influence on the future work opportunities that are available for you.

The reasons for a career change vary, and a good place to start is by honestly understanding your motives for leaving medicine. Only after you formulate a clear understanding of why you want to make a change will you be able to evaluate the best future alternatives for yourself. Do you feel fascinated

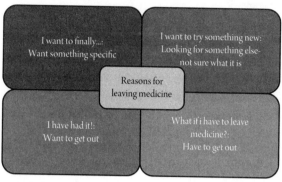

Figure 1.1 Reasons for leaving medicine.

by another professional pursuit or are you primarily driven by your desire to avoid unpleasant aspects of your work as a doctor? The appeal of a new goal may be strong or weak, specific or vague, as can the need to leave medicine. See Figure 1.1. Most likely, as a physician, your goals in considering a different job involve more than one of the following categories and possibly even a mixture of all four. As you begin to recognize where you fit in the following section (arranged from a strong interest in a specific alternative career, to a vague interest in doing something different, to a vague dislike of medicine, and finally to a strong need to get out of medicine), you can gain assurance in knowing that you are not the only good doctor considering the pursuit of a career path outside of clinical practice and that your reasons are not atypical. When you begin to appreciate more clearly which features of medicine you may still be drawn to, you will become better equipped to evaluate which characteristics of an alternative field are appealing enough to motivate you to devote your time and energy to.

The Four Main Reasons for Leaving Medicine

I Want to Finally …

In order to be a great doctor a person has to have the ability to master a large volume of specialized medical knowledge, to apply it to serious real-life situations, and to make the right decisions for the best patient outcome at the right time. A doctor also has to be able to calm people in their time of need and to make patients, other physicians, and everyone involved in the patient's care comfortable. You have been trained in high-stress situations, and you have the capacity to help others understand what is happening now and what to expect next. You likely enjoy numerous qualities of the daily work of treating patients when they are sick.

But what if you have other talents or interests that you would like to devote more time to? What if there is another field that you are fascinated by but have not had the time or opportunity to explore? For instance, after training and working as a physician, you may now want to become involved in medical device development, health policy, develop real estate, or pursue your talent as a musician. What if you have dabbled in your nonclinical interest? Perhaps you want to start a business, either related to the medical field or completely unrelated to healthcare. What if you have contemplated working in another field and you know that it will require a serious time commitment to do it right? You may have a nagging sense that, while you spend the majority of your time and energy working as a doctor, you are missing out on engaging in something else that is genuinely exciting and interesting for you. Perhaps, for example, you have occasionally taught and advised students, only to discover that you want to meaningfully expand that type of work. Your rational acknowledgment that you like medicine, but that you want to focus and dedicate your time and effort to another pursuit, is a valid reason to carefully evaluate the big step of getting started in a new career.

Your practice of medicine itself may have sparked another interest that you want to become involved with on a more committed level. A young ophthalmologist from the East Coast who used implants in surgery became fascinated by the details of implant materials and composition. As he became more familiar with the mechanical aspects of implanted devices, he realized that he wanted to work on improving biomedical devices for improved patient outcomes, even outside of his specialty of ophthalmology. As a young physician, he found himself initially unable to obtain employment in the biomedical field until after he attained a few years of clinical experience. Recognizing that he was more interested in the manufacturing aspects of ophthalmologic devices, he remained in medical practice until he was able to secure a satisfying full-time position in his area of interest. As in this example, many doctors have noticed a significant deficit in the available treatment or management of medical conditions. In order to devote more time to effectively filling this gap, a physician might leave clinical practice to work full-time on a solution to an unsolved problem in the health care field. Doctors typically tend to be very committed and oriented toward high-quality work. Some physicians feel that pursuing parallel work endeavors can result in cutting corners, which many consider unacceptable.

Alternately, there are doctors who do not want to give up clinical practice because they enjoy it, yet want to figure out how to create a customized blend of clinical practice and an additional professional activity. Glenn Graham, MD, PhD, a neurologist from New Mexico, practiced at the Veterans Administration and University of New Mexico Hospitals for over fifteen years. He was involved in policy and advocacy, when he realized that he found this type of work to be even more interesting than what he did on a day-to-day basis. He eventually decided to pursue a job in health policy with the Department of Veterans Affairs so that he could be more effective in guiding healthcare delivery. He says that he might not have been willing to give up full-time clinical medicine twenty (or even ten) years ago, echoing many physicians' opinions that professional interests may evolve with time and experience.

Similarly, time may play a role in the decision that some very competent doctors make in deciding to take time off or to work part-time in order to devote more time to the job of being fathers or mothers while their children are young. It was very common for young female physicians in the past to feel that their early academic success had ironically served to penalize them to a life with limited and demanding work options. Many women physicians who are now near retirement speak of being treated by peers almost as if they were disabled whenever they disclosed a pregnancy or mentioned that they had a sick child at home. These physicians expressed regret at missing family events for the purpose of appearing perfectly dedicated at work. On a similar note, the media portrayed an exaggerated dichotomy between working mothers and stay-at-home mothers in the 1990s, accentuating the personal insecurities associated with either choice and effectively instigating some mothers to dig in their heels as they allowed themselves to be strictly defined either as career women or stay-at-home moms. Fortunately, the mommy wars of the 1990s are long gone, and many parents of young children now feel confident in making career adjustments that allow a balance of priorities, letting go of rigid definitions. Confining labels have largely given way to recognition of fluidity in work arrangements for many professionals. While many physicians I have spoken with have been able to excellently balance their full-time clinical work with their family lives, some have made the choice, even temporarily, to cut back on professional hours.

However, despite societal recognition in many professions that there are more choices than the extremes of intensely long work days versus not working at all, as physician overhead costs rise, while reimbursement falls, and time-consuming form-filling increases, it can be difficult, from a practical standpoint, for physicians to economically sustain part-time clinical work even in light of broad-minded attitudes about work flexibility. Furthermore, doctors in certain specialties have concerns that expressing the desire to work part-time may diminish credibility among peers. This realization prompts many physicians to reevaluate their career choice and to look for other options besides direct patient care.

These motivations are included in the strong interest category because they are endeavors besides clinical medicine that may attract doctors who *do not dislike* the practice of medicine, but instead want to make choices based on realistic time availability for several attractive, yet demanding goals.

You may have decided that it is the right time to make a pivotal decision about your undeveloped professional or personal interest that has been on the back burner. You can use the concrete facts and information presented here to construct a time frame for initiating and following through with your plan for a new professional route that will make you happy. You could be interested in another goal outside of medical practice, and while confident of your abilities, you may wish to figure out if your non clinical professional interest can provide a suitable income or if your plan will be too costly. Many physicians have non-patient-care professional goals and have been unable to figure out how to make their aspirations work from a practical standpoint. As you evaluate the important elements involved, you can begin to take the essential steps to achieving your objectives as you learn how other physicians have achieved their goals in similar situations.

I Want to Try Something New

What if you are happy being a physician? Does that mean that you would not want to explore another field? What if you feel that it is getting monotonous for you? Can you explore the world of business, education, or technology? Can you do something creative? Often, doctors want to try something new and feel that they have practiced medicine "enough." Perhaps you are unlike the doctors who have a specific professional passion in mind. Maybe, in contrast, you have a vague nonmedical interest or feel ambivalent about medicine. You might feel that while clinical medicine was a fine job for you, it was only a step along the way to a new season in your professional path. You may view your medical background as part of the foundation for your career development rather than as defining your whole career.

It is not uncommon for bright young people to enter into the field of medicine simply as a way to go with the flow. It is often an assumption that promising students, if they are able to achieve the difficult accomplishment of getting accepted into medical school, should not decline such a prestigious opportunity. However, some may actually feel indifference toward the medical profession, a profession that attracts competitive students who would have had the capability to achieve meaningful success in a number of other fields as well. Medicine may be okay for you, but not exactly the right fit.

In the book *Free Agent Nation*, Daniel Pink describes an increasing trend of professionals in different fields changing jobs much more frequently than in the past. From my discussions with many physicians, I am learning that some doctors, like other professionals, may aspire to a well-rounded professional experience and varied expertise in addition to the specialized proficiency attained in medical training and practice.

It is possible that many areas of interest have caught your attention over the years. Perhaps you have an affinity toward journalism, economics, community planning, or public health. You may be looking for the tools to help you investigate your nonclinical employment prospects as a physician, in terms of financial practicality, job availability, and job security, before embarking on a time-consuming job search.

While you might enjoy your clinical work, you may have become captivated by how another aspect of medical business works. A physical medicine and rehabilitation specialist who spent years treating patients with disabilities in the hospital setting became involved in writing disability guidelines on a part-time basis. She noticed that she liked the setting, teamwork approach, and interaction with colleagues more with this type of work. She eventually left her clinical job to work full-time doing disability evaluations and writing guidelines, not because she specifically relished writing disability directives, but because she preferred her new work environment to the hospital setting.

Some doctors quickly work their way up the hierarchical ladder to leadership roles. Given that these positions are subject to significant turnover, they can be relatively short-term posts. It is common for physicians in leadership positions to relocate frequently. Yet, at times, relocation may be impractical. Therefore, the conclusion of a leadership position may serve as a transitional hinge for a doctor who has an inclination for exploring nonclinical possibilities.

You could also reflect on the fact that, if you wish for another job but still do not know what you are looking for, there are likely important *characteristics* and aspects of professional life that you feel are lacking from your current daily work arrangement. Are you searching for the opportunity to be creative, to develop technology, or to have a role in problem solving on an organizational level? These are important considerations, as several possible careers may be attractive and suitable for you, as long as they encompass the *features* that you are looking for. Chapter 4 explores diverse professional qualities relevant to physicians to help you in assessing what you are looking for, and why you may be restless or dissatisfied with clinical medicine. If you know that you have a general idea that you want to switch careers but you need to solidify your goals, Chapter 5, which contains descriptions of nonclinical work opportunities for doctors and their vastly different features, can help you judge which options fulfill your individual criteria. If you have a vague professional goal, you can find a way for this vague dissatisfaction to realistically translate into a viable job. There exist a great deal of opportunities for doctors in the fields of industry, science, business, communication, and public health that do not enjoy a direct route from medical school or residency training. Yet while the route is not well paved, it certainly exists and is not difficult to find.

I Have Had It!

It is no secret that being a doctor can be frustrating on a day-to-day basis. The most well recognized frustration is the long hours. Since 2002, The

Accreditation Council for Graduate Medical Education (which is responsible for the accreditation of post-MD medical training programs in the United States) has mandatorily cut residency training to an eighty-hour maximum workweek. Until that time, many residency programs required much more than eighty hours of work per week. And, typically, that work requires the resident to be in three places at once, and to go home and read during time off in order to be knowledgeable about patients' medical conditions, in addition to doing well on tests and examinations.

Practicing physicians are formally relieved of a minimum or maximum number of allowed work hours. But the nature of caring for sick patients makes weekends and holidays an essential component of the job forever. Whether self-employed or a hospital or institutional employee, it is principally a physician's direct patient care productivity that must bring in enough income to cover all administrative, management, and staff salaries, expenditures for abiding with mandates and regulations, building and equipment expenses, operating costs, and medical malpractice insurance payments. The high cost of overhead, especially in large metropolitan cities, leaves little room for reasonable work hours. While you may enjoy the work of being a doctor, the necessary time commitment and volume of work required to break even can lead to burnout and dissatisfaction with your job and your life.

As reimbursement rates have fallen, employed physicians are often forced by hospital systems to accept patient appointments at shorter intervals in order to maintain a revenue flow. At the same time, documentation requirements have become more extensive, the preauthorization process for diagnostic tests, treatments, and referrals has become more time-consuming, and checklists add documentation time while they encroach on patient care time during a scheduled appointment. Efforts to improve healthcare cost and delivery often result in new mandates, such as outcomes parameters and required worksheets, without corresponding funding. All of these changes do not necessarily help the physician to understand the patient's medical complaint or emotional state or to explain the diagnosis and plan, much less answer patient questions. For physicians, who may lose track of their noble goals, idealism can be crushed, leaving many doctors wondering if it is possible to maintain integrity while accommodating the outside controls that restrict medical care.

When it comes to income, some doctors feel dissatisfied with their perceived low income, when compared to peers in fields such as banking, law, or business. It is important to note, however, that changes in the economy have been known to destabilize such fields as much as, or even more than, medicine. In contrast, other doctors feel awkward about the popular notion that doctors earn *too* much money. This can be a difficult adjustment, particularly if family members or friends harbor resentment toward you or feel inadequate themselves.

The lifestyle can be stressful for many physicians. I once heard a pediatrician joke that parents bring their sick children to the doctor and expect, in return, a new and improved version of that child (in comparison to before the illness). And every doctor has had the exasperating experience of dealing with a patient who really doesn't seem to want to get better. While only a tiny percentage of patients have unrealistic, or even dishonest expectations, the negativity and the ever-present threat of predatory malpractice lawsuits can bring a tense flavor into what could have been an otherwise gratifying job.

Colleagues can be competitive. Unfortunately, a hallmark of some doctors' personalities is what is referred to as "the blame game." These doctors are few and far between, and everybody in the hospital or clinic recognizes this type of personality. But the dysfunctional physician who, when unsure of how to approach a clinical problem, brashly blames a patient's condition inaccurately on another doctor or hospital, contributes to an atmosphere of defensiveness and anxiety among patients and staff alike. Additionally, restructured requirements for maintenance of certification, which is a prerequisite for hospital privileges and insurance authorization, are often expensive and time-consuming.

I have heard so many unsolicited stories from physicians about insurance hassles. Doctors all too frequently complain of denials, underpayment, late payments, incorrect payments, patients who thought they were covered but weren't, conditions that used to be covered but aren't, guidelines that bafflingly change, guidelines that are not medically sound, bills that were not received, and the worst of all: AUDITS.

One particular story really stood out for me because I know many physicians who have been very intimidated by similar situations. Judah Lindenberg, MD, a neurologist, had a particularly organized billing system. He received THE letter. Medicare told him that he had overbilled and refused to pay. He knew that he had been detailed and careful with his documentation. He reviewed his patient charts and billing just to be sure. He had made no billing errors. He resubmitted the bills, but received no response. He could not foot the bill for an attorney, nor did he want to pay the unjust and costly fine.

He contacted his state and local medical societies, who provided an ombudsman to help him with the matter. After numerous letters, faxes, e-mails, and hours and hours of clerical work, he was finally vindicated. This was a fourteen-month struggle when all was said and done. Medicare finally paid back the bills they owed him. He was unfortunately unable to succeed in getting them to pay his months and months of overdue bills with interest, or to compensate him for his wasted time. But he can still continue to be a great doctor. It was difficult and unfair, but he overcame the obstacle and moved on.

We can, and should, work to overcome unfair problems. But, understandably, the process of fighting such aggravation is often too time-consuming, intimidating, expensive, and emotionally taxing for most physicians. Some physicians fear the threat of medical malpractice or billing audits to a degree that is disabling. The strain of billing audits and medical malpractice lawsuits can contribute to physician divorce, substance abuse, and sadly, in some cases, suicide. In fact, for some doctors, the emotional devastation caused by medical malpractice lawsuits and audits can last for generations. Becoming a lawyer is a common coping mechanism for young adult offspring of doctors who have had to face significant lawsuits. As a physician yourself, you may be dealing with a sense of unfairness and helplessness regarding a lawsuit. Can you learn to deal in a more effective and efficient way with these fears? Do you want to? Can you pinpoint the areas that make your job unpleasant and change them? Or are the stresses and feelings of burnout so bad that you are ready to move on?

Given the state of healthcare, there are many obstacles to being a good doctor. The excessive documentation requirements on one hand, contrasted with denials of patient care on the other hand, and what often seem like arbitrary rules, make providing good care feel like a target that doctors aim for *despite* the barriers in the system, not with the support of the system. There are higher expectations of physicians from multiple entities, less physician control of clinical patient management, lower reimbursement, more bureaucracy, more public mistrust of healthcare institutions, and little support for physicians as they try to keep up with so many new rules and regulations. While many of the changes in medicine must have been well intentioned, they have had a burdensome effect on the practice of medicine. Many physicians have expressed "I have worked so hard, for so long, trying to help people and all I get is pay cuts, watching my back, everybody trying to regulate my work without helping, and I have had it!"

A very important question is raised, however: is the system bad enough that you no longer want to continue the uphill battle to be a great doctor? Perhaps you cannot envision a desirable future for yourself in the medical field anymore. Perhaps you feel that you are struggling just to keep your head above water. Certainly, any doctor would agree that there are features of medical practice that no one would ever wish for. There are probably some aspects of clinical practice that are not quite what you expected, and many doctors feel that there are too many players waiting to capitalize on any perceived misstep on the part of a vulnerable physician. And if it weren't for the satisfaction of being able to have such a positive effect on the health of our fellow human beings, few would remain in the medical field. Of course, there are struggles in every type of work. As a neurologist, I heard so many patients talk about real, heartbreaking anxieties stemming from their jobs, that it helped me cope with my own irritation at redundant paperwork and the diminishing control that I had over my patients' care. And after I left my clinical practice due to the time commitment associated with my utilization review job, I decided to continue to see patients part-time as a volunteer neurologist in a free clinic. The human aspect of medicine, seeing sick people, or hearing the stories of the unemployed and uninsured, is likely what allows so many doctors to put aside the numerous shortcomings of the healthcare system and persevere.

Most physicians who feel that they want to get out of medicine rather than feeling drawn to something else initially entered medicine with altruistic intentions but find that they are unable to make the excessive sacrifices necessary to practice good medicine. Anthony Valenti, MD, who cofounded and co-owns a successful telemedicine business, believes that most doctors go into medicine for good reasons, but he encounters many who feel that they want to get out of medicine because there are conflicts between how they want to practice based on integrity and the realities of the job. While a career as a physician has been attainable for you, perhaps it is simply not a good fit for your personality at this time. If your fundamental motive for looking into alternative career options is that you are unhappy with your clinical practice, the only thing standing in your way of moving on may be figuring out the details of how to do so.

What if I Have to Leave Medicine?

This is every physician's greatest fear when it comes to medicine. It trumps concerns about salary, malpractice, and even insurance reimbursements. It is one thing to be accused of not being a great physician but another to actually BE less than great. This dreadful fear is more common early in a physician's career, but may continue. Medical students typically begin medical school and within a few months are sent in to interview patients and to select and support a diagnosis. Residents take call with responsibilities for many unstable patients and are routinely reminded (not necessarily kindly) that their performance was lacking.

In reality, medical students and residents are the lucky ones. They have teachers, mentors, senior residents, attending physicians, and a whole system in place for teaching, evaluation, and even quality assurance. Yes, sometimes the process for correcting shortcomings can be insensitive and indiscreet. Medicine, like many worthwhile endeavors in life, does undeniably require accountability, responsibility, thick skin, an open mind, and hard work.

As practicing physicians, we no longer have the harsh criticism and direction of medical school and residency to fall back on. You are responsible. The consequences of being less than perfect are severe: poor patient outcomes, fewer patients, malpractice suits, and hospital privilege restrictions. Continuing Medical Education (CME) is available and is required by most states for maintenance of licensure. But, while continuing to review and update knowledge is critical, what really matters is clinical judgment and procedural skill. I believe that as medicine continues to evolve and improve, more attention may one day finally be directed toward worthwhile improvements, such as developing better systems for continued evaluation, mentoring, and supplementation of skills, as well as partnerships for clinical decision-making and more systematic attention dedicated to preemptive error reduction.

If your goal at one point was to be a great doctor, yet you think that you are merely satisfactory, there will be a crucial point when you will need to evaluate whether you still want to be a practicing clinical doctor. You should not give up on the goal that inspired you in the past simply because you are attaining it at a slower pace. Malcolm Gladwell, in his book *Outliers*, illustrates how expertise is primarily attained through practice and experience, rather than pure talent. Given that you have already received the formal validation that you can become an excellent doctor, there is certainly no reason to believe that excellence as a practicing physician is an unattainable goal for you.

It could be helpful to look into courses or seminars in your field. Everyone has to continue to learn. The "best" doctors at the "best" hospitals often hold department conferences to discuss challenging cases. This option may not be available in some hospitals or small practices. Yet, even in such situations, a, doctor can initiate second opinions by sending challenging patients to a well-respected colleague. You can call other physicians for advice, and, after some time, you will trust and improve your own clinical skills and judgment. Doctors should not be afraid to view other doctors as partners rather than judges.

You can take a more significant course of action and obtain additional formal training as well. There has been a proliferation of medical knowledge over the past several decades, with resulting improvement in healthcare capabilities. Many doctors find it difficult to know everything about everything. There is certainly nothing wrong with admitting that and in obtaining additional or updated training after having practiced for a while. It can be a revitalizing experience to supplement and update your medical skills with a fellowship or workshop and to obtain objective direction and feedback from other physicians in the setting of a training program.

Another reason that doctors may have to change career direction is health concerns. Physicians treat patients with disabilities and health problems, often recommending work modification for patients. Yet, when physicians become moderately disabled, more often than not, they do not want to quit working altogether. Physicians who suffer from disability or illness have a need to continue to earn an income, but may not be able to perform the intense work of patient care medicine. In fact, even when these situations occur in the context of financial stability or near retirement, MDs often prefer to work at a job that is less demanding than clinical medicine, rather than not to work at all. A busy solo-practicing dentist in the Midwest was diagnosed with cancer. During his own medical treatment, he experienced significant fatigue and nausea. He chose to supervise dental students during their clinical rotations during his hiatus from practice in order to remain in the dental field while maintaining a flexible, relaxed schedule to suit his health needs.

In contrast to physicians who choose to leave medicine to pursue something else, these doctors *must* decrease work responsibilities, not because of time, but because of issues such as health concerns or professional considerations. The drive to continue to make a difference and to learn new things, even when unable to work at full force, is one of the many reasons that doctors look for nontraditional work opportunities.

The Crucial Question

The central question at this stage is: do you still wish to be a doctor? This is a fundamental question that you must ask yourself because, at this point, your next step will require a great deal of hard work and self-discipline, regardless of your decision. While this book is written as a guide to help doctors navigate a transition from traditional medical practice to a genuinely desirable alternative, I do not embrace a value judgment that remaining in medicine or leaving medicine is a better decision. My descriptions of some of the negative aspects of medical practice are undeniable facts that have been repeated by numerous physicians, and are not value judgments. It is important to acknowledge the negative facts and to understand them, knowing that your future options will inevitably, in some way, incorporate an acceptance of, or a purposeful attempt to alter, the current day-to-day frustrations that all healthcare providers and patients face.

If you decide to remain in clinical medicine, you need to reevaluate your priorities and construct a plan to change the frustrating aspects of your job. I had felt frustrated about the repeated health insurance denials for radiology tests that I requested for my patients. After numerous unpleasant phone calls, I finally decided to get to know more about the other side of the story. I was able to convince the CEO of the utilization management company to hire me to help with setting guidelines and reviewing appeals from other physicians. It was certainly a useful learning experience for me as I learned to appreciate that insurance companies deal with many requests for unnecessary, incorrect, and redundant diagnostic tests. I also learned how to more efficiently order imaging tests for my own patients, and I used this information to help my fellow physicians order tests more effectively too.

If you can't stand coding hassles but love seeing patients, it could help to take a course on billing and coding. This can allow you to become an expert. Then you can even teach a class yourself! Identify and master the precise challenge that is troubling you and get that frustration out of your system. Are you working too

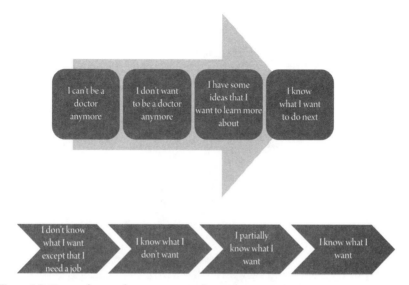

Figure 1.2 Do you know what you want to do next?

much? Maybe you can take a closer look at your collections and try to improve your collection rates with better follow-up or staff incentives. Perhaps, then, you can afford to hire a part-time physician assistant or a moonlighting doctor to help take some of your workload off. If the small changes in these types of scenarios would be enough to provide you with fulfillment as a medical doctor, then maybe you do not need a drastic career switch. You can continue to be a great doctor, and be content with your career and your life.

However, for many of the doctors I have spoken to, careful reflection about the career of medicine marks a resolution to change gears. Whether your motivation for leaving medicine is burnout, disillusionment, or a longing to finally start your own web design company, you will need to work hard. It is advantageous to evaluate the balance of factors involved in your decision and your realistic chances of achieving whatever it is that is professionally motivating you. See Figure 1.2.

If you want to pursue another interest, you must address your feelings about leaving medicine, and whether you still expect to hold on to some aspects of being a doctor. Weighing how much you are drawn to a new career versus how much you enjoy practicing medicine plays a large role in deciding your next step. You are fortunate if your reason for leaving is that you are pulled in several directions, because you already know that you have good options.

If you wish to or have to leave medicine, it is important to remember that almost any position you take in the future, even outside of medicine, will require a degree of accountability, and will come with the risks of stress and criticism. You have many alternatives if you do not think that remaining in clinical practice

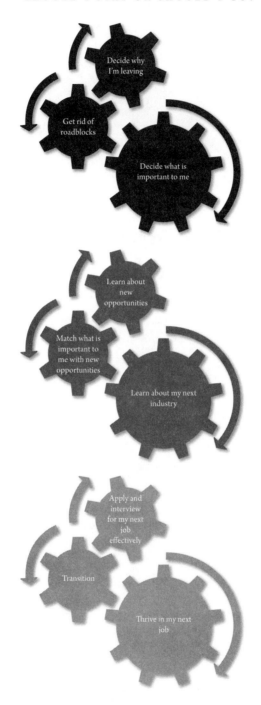

Figure 1.3 Steps to your next career.

is the best choice for you at this time. If you are unsure what to do next, the following chapters can to help you determine which aspects of professional life are important to you and how to choose your next step, as well as how to effectively make the shift. Definitely, in this time of transformations in the healthcare landscape, there are a variety of worthwhile choices that will suit your skills and personality, allowing you to make a productive transition regardless of your current situation.

Many physicians have chosen different paths, and for different reasons, with variable continued clinical involvement. All have had unique experiences, with few role models in the nonclinical arena. They all have had to make some compromises and have used the framework provided by medicine to add to the medical field or to the world exercising a different approach than what was taught in training. You can use some of the advice and experience of other doctors as you construct your own career path using a method that is best suited for you. See Figure 1.3.

The Metamorphosis of Medicine and How It Affects You

When a physician is in the process of shifting professional direction, career stage can have an influence on the available options. Experienced and midcareer physicians have been confronted with modifications in the healthcare environment that may contribute to a change of heart about continuing to practice medicine, even for doctors who were previously satisfied with medical practice. On the other hand, while young physicians or residents and medical students do not reminisce about the "good old days" when they begin to encounter what medical work entails, they must use this time to evaluate whether they can handle the modern challenges of being a doctor as well as whether they want to.

There is an overall transformation in the structure of the medical field as well as a change in the attitude of doctors. It is impossible to determine which came first, but they influence each other in positive ways as well as negative. As society's esteem for physicians lessens, physicians themselves want to lead more "normal" lives, often electing to work more predictable hours than physicians in years past while accepting increasing regulation. As doctors view medicine more as "just a job" than in the past, more nonphysician participants begin to make important medical decisions for patients.

Medicine Is Changing

If you are a young doctor, you have a different outlook and set of concerns regarding the medical profession than more senior physicians. As you enter the world of medicine, you will, no doubt, realize that, for better or for worse, you will not have the same career as doctors of previous generations. Because of the current healthcare atmosphere, new physicians have a number of advantages both in medical practice and in alternative medical careers. More experienced physicians have a different set of advantages when it comes to traditional medical work and nonclinical medical routes, because they have had the opportunity to establish themselves as experts in various aspects of the medical field.

In clinical practice itself there are new features that discourage older, more seasoned physicians, which will, fortunately, not be as challenging for younger physicians or for those in training. Medicine has evolved in such a way that, on the road to a better healthcare system, certain growing pains have made the current structure exasperating for patients and for veteran physicians alike. However, in my opinion, the undesirable side effects of curing the healthcare system have nearly peaked, and future physicians might enjoy the gains of the recent advancements and, hopefully simultaneously, a more streamlined healthcare structure providing a better ability to do the job.

For example, while electronic medical records can allow easier management of patient information than in the past, experienced physicians must adapt to the inconvenience of learning a new system, as well as absorbing the steep financial cost of implementing new technology. This can lead to frustration for highly competent, focused physicians who are required to comply with new computer systems that can take seemingly endless hours to become familiar with. Additionally, obtaining important patient care information from these new systems can create time-consuming roadblocks for those who, as an illustration, may not have the necessary password handy in order to retrieve information. Imagine the annoyance for a physician, who, in recent memory, could simply hold a chart and look up relevant patient information in a predictable location. As a young doctor, who is part of the generation accustomed to the dramatic, relatively recent, technological advancements, you do not look at computer systems as potential mystery boxes, holding critical reports that you often cannot access, but rather as useful tools that you cannot live without, and that never leave you dumbfounded.

Similarly, over the past ten to fifteen years, physician documentation requirements have become more and more closely tied to billing. It is often lamented by physicians that documentation requirements are sometimes irrelevant to patient care. This can be cumbersome for experienced physicians, who have spent years using documentation to enhance patient care and thorough health provider communication rather than to complete health insurance forms, which may not reflect medically relevant applicability. Because you are training at a time when healthcare has already changed in this way, you will not have to adjust your documentation patterns to suit new regulations.

Doctors often note that new physician ranking and outcomes measures, accessed easily by patients, can be unrelated to MD qualifications or actual performance. Recently, the task of staying on top of ranking, found on numerous websites, has added time and administrative cost for physicians and hospitals as well. As a young physician, such measures may not seem so foreign or upsetting to you, as it has become commonplace for consumers in many industries to anonymously rate every type of product. However, the classification of physician care as a product and the patient as consumer can be deeply offensive to doctors of previous generations.

Current times require professionals, such as physicians, to conduct work in a more transparent way than in the past. While one of the great benefits of this transparency in medicine is that it can effectively work to prevent wasteful or duplicitous billing practices, one of the more recent side effects is that it can leave your practice vulnerable to evaluation by many who are not properly skilled to do so. Physicians have been subject to transparency, while many other players in the healthcare system have not. A family doctor with a public health degree comments that this unbalanced situation will undoubtedly change, as transparency has become customary from more and more industries as they are expected by the public to operate in an open and legitimate manner. The contagious effect could eventually reach the whole healthcare system, allowing coverage of medical services, medical billing, and collections to become easier to decipher for medical institutions, patients, and employers.

Reimbursement rates for doctor's work have been stagnant for some physicians and declining for others. In the meantime, the cost of living typically increases. What each individual defines as a high or low salary is remarkably variable, and that personal viewpoint is the consequence of years of contributing factors. But most people would agree that for any typical person, *declining* reimbursement for the same amount of work is cause for stress and anxiety. Given that, if you are a new physician, you have no doubt heard the buzz that physician's salaries are declining, and possibly poised to decline even more, you most likely have not taken on the same burden of financial commitments, either on a personal or professional level, reflective of past physician earnings, that some older physicians have.

Many experienced physicians have to adjust their practices, as they are unable to continue to afford support staff, save as expected for retirement, or even sustain a viable practice. A well-respected private practice surgeon with whom I spoke explains that this reality has caused his practice to close shop. He states that he feels fortunate to have been able to securely dissolve his practice and retire early, but that he has concerns about colleagues who are currently stuck without a viable exit strategy. As with the previously mentioned concerns, if you are new to medicine, you are entering medicine with more of a clean slate, when you have not made financial commitments or hired employees that will have to go if your situation becomes unsustainable.

It is important to note, however, that just as the above changes in healthcare have been stressful for some senior physicians, many doctors attribute their success in large part on their willingness to adapt to change. Some established

Table 2.1 **Changes in Medicine**

Do you view these modifications positively or negatively?
Some doctors view these and other changes as aggravations, other doctors view them as innovative changes.
Increased Documentation Requirements
Increased Preauthorization Guidelines
Electronic Medical Records
Outcomes Measures
Evidence-Based Medicine
Physician Ranking
Increased Patient Privacy
Lower Physician Compensation
Payer Control of Prescription Drug Costs
Prescription Medication Commercials for the Public
Accountable Care Organization Proposals
Residency Work Hour Limits
Increased Hospitalist Care
Drop-in Clinics
Concierge Medical Care
Health Insurance Mandates for the Public

physicians in clinical practice have taken the time, well after completion of training, to focus on learning to use new interventional or diagnostic technology or to master new developments in medicine. On the other hand, a surgeon from the Midwest explains that when that her senior partners failed to learn updated innovative surgical techniques, this led the hospital to recruit another surgeon, causing a significant financial impact in the group. See Table 2.1.

The popular 1998 book *Who Moved My Cheese*, by Spencer Johnson, MD, describes the allegorical story of a group of fictional mice that have to figure out what to do when their cheese is no longer in its expected place. Several mice insist on remaining in their place, hopeful that the cheese will reappear. A few other mice however, take the approach of searching for more cheese in different places. Sadly, the mice that feared leaving the traditional cheese spot were wrong, and cheese did not reappear. On the other hand, the mice that looked around for more cheese, while unsuccessful at first, eventually found more cheese and also learned that they could overcome cheese scarcity if such a dire situation were to recur again.

Similarly, professionals, MDs or otherwise, who are able to adapt as necessary are more satisfied and successful. Medicine is benefiting from great advances in technology. On a large scale, this has contributed to the increase in healthcare costs nationally. Put simply, when there are more available high technology treatments, they must cost more money. When patients live longer and survive illnesses that previously were untreatable, most likely the price of medication alone will cause that patient to cost the healthcare system more than if the patient had died a decade earlier. This irrefutably positive outcome is one of the causes of the increased cost of healthcare and, as a result, the cost-saving measures and costly bureaucracy. The physician, of any age and with any level of experience, who can adapt and respond to the changes in the healthcare environment, whether they were wisely thought out changes or not, is, like the brave mouse, able to survive despite changes. Medicine is transforming and it will continue to transform. Where medicine is heading, no one knows for sure. The question of who actually controls the cheese will continue to be a markedly complex one, but the resourceful doctor who can continue to locate it, either in clinical medicine or in any nontraditional field, will ultimately survive. It is interesting to note that the author of *Who Moved My Cheese* is a physician.

Kevin Chin, MD, a radiologist from the West Coast, has worked in telemedicine for about ten years. He had heard about telemedicine when he was a practicing radiologist and wanted to become part of the emerging field in part to proactively prevent his skills from becoming obsolete. He believes that his timing was right, as technological advancements allowed him to enter the field of telemedicine at a stage when there was tremendous growth, offering him many opportunities. As several other physicians have mentioned, the frequent changes in healthcare regulation, and an evolving market for certain services, has a significant impact on professional opportunities. He found his position through word of mouth through mutual acquaintances of the then fledgling company founders.

He explains that, while the exponential growth in telemedicine for radiology services has stabilized, telemedicine has been more recently growing in other medical specialties, such as pathology, neonatology fetal monitoring, intensive care monitoring, and echocardiogram reading. He says that the primary need is based on the fact that small hospitals, which can only support one or a few specialists due to low volume, are often unable to obtain enough on-call coverage to cover twenty-four hours per day, seven days a week. This frequently necessitates outsourcing for specialized services. Physicians may have to respond to budding developments in healthcare delivery by learning new skills in order to prevent being left behind or outdated professionally. These new skills can involve direct patient care or a command of nontraditional skills in order to have an enduring impact on the healthcare system.

As you continue in your career, whether in direct patient care or not, you should be reassured that while you adapt to the changes in healthcare, the healthcare industry is responding to unproductive developments more so in recent years than in the past. The Texas Medical Association has taken steps to develop a toolkit to help physicians challenge unfair rankings. Health insurers have not been required to publish guidelines for covered conditions and treatments, but recently Fair Health, a nonprofit organization, has made strides in ensuring fairness and transparency in out-of-network reimbursement by assisting consumers estimate the out-of-pocket costs they may be responsible for paying if they use out-of-network care. Physicians have recently noted a completely new phenomenon of health insurance company surveys aimed at improving physician satisfaction, a concept that was unheard of as recently as a few years ago.

Advantages for the Experienced Doctor

Experienced physicians who want to change careers also have great advantages attained over the years of practicing medicine. See Table 2.2. Undoubtedly medicine is fluctuating, while you may be changing and possibly experiencing an evolution of your own priorities. The ability to effectively adjust to unpredictable developments that can impact your day-to-day work or to shape and influence the developments in healthcare yourself can turn a frustrating job situation into a gratifying one.

Physicians who have practiced medicine for several years enjoy the benefits of having already created a foundation of know-how in the healthcare industry. On the path to another facet of healthcare, experienced physicians have a background that can be used as leverage during the shift into an alternative career. Because of this, older physicians often enter a new nonclinical career at higher positions than less experienced MDs.

A physician specialized in primary care works as a high-level administrator and states that one of her inspirational triggers occurred when she worked for a large hospital that had been trying for years to compete with a nearby hospital for market share. After her employer of twenty years invested several million dollars for the guidance of a management consulting company, the hospital laid off office employees and nursing staff in order to save money, later replacing them with temporary employees instead. The hospital also changed its name from the equivalent of "Children's Hospital" to the equivalent of "Hospital for Children," incurring the costs of making new signs, and changing the name on all hospital publications. At the time, she was also being pressured to see more patients in order to increase revenue. She was in danger of having a salary cut due to patient "no shows." Instead of giving in to discouragement, she decided

Table 2.2 **the Level of Experience and Stage of a Medical Career can Impact the Possibilities Available to a Physician When Making a Transition.**

Advantages for Experienced Doctors	Advantages for Young Doctors
Confidence	Humble
Wisdom	More objective about medicine
Credibility	More time to establish experience in alternative fields
Experience	Learn new things easily
Impressive CV	Can change direction
Already have networks in the healthcare field	Can use medical school and residency resources
Financial Stability	Fewer financial entanglements

to take another approach. She says that twenty years of clinical practice made her "far too old to be disillusioned." Having gained confidence, wisdom, and experience from her clinical work as well as from her observations of systematic decisions, she leveraged her experience to find a position as an administrator in her own hospital, using her skills to focus on fostering patient loyalty and satisfaction.

I'm Just Getting Started and I Already Don't Like It—Is It Me or Is It Medicine?

If you are a medical student or resident, you are facing a unique time in your career. Regardless of your age, you are only at the beginning of a long future as a doctor. But maybe you have wondered whether you really want to remain in medicine. It is very common, at this stage, to have doubts and reservations about your future career as a physician. See Figure 2.1.

You have worked hard to get to this point, and, instead of taking a respite after intense preparation for especially challenging medical school entrance examinations, applications, and interviews, you immediately have even more work thrust upon you in medical school and residency. Even if you went to a prominent undergraduate university, the competition that you face among your current physician-in-training colleagues is quite intense. The environment in medical school and residency may cause even the highest achieving students to feel shockingly average among their peers for the very first time in their lives.

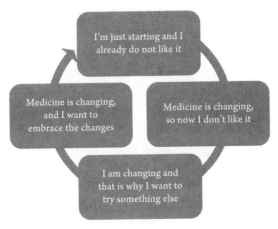

Figure 2.1 What is changing?

However, if we fast-forward to the future, physicians who have completed training do not express regret about the intensity of training. Surely, a medical education does not close any doors for the future. It is rare, even unheard of, to hear a physician comment, "I resent that I worked as hard as I did," or "I wish I had not studied that challenging material." Most doctors recognize that in the United States, despite the bureaucracy associated with healthcare delivery, it is good physicians who work hard and persevere who have made our healthcare the best in the world.

It can be difficult to determine whether as a young physician, your interest in leaving medicine is caused by diving into a new kind of stress or whether medicine is truly the wrong field for you.

Stress

Being a doctor entails a new type of responsibility. Young physicians in training must learn how to cope with the anxiety associated with taking care of sick patients, and the fact that there are real, often life-and-death consequences to every clinical decision. While you entered medical school to learn under supervision how to help sick patients, it quickly became apparent that the decisions concerning when to intervene and how to intervene would soon depend on you. Several prominent physicians revealed an initial lack of confidence regarding this serious responsibility. A pulmonologist who has traveled to many countries in disaster situations, and has had to figure out how to deal with novel medical problems, such as learning vascular surgery and how to perform C-sections *while* in the field, humbly explains that she was initially apprehensive about the prospect of taking care of patients as an intern. In fact, this modest realization of the seriousness of a physician's clinical work eventually dawns on every doctor, and may be more profound if it occurs later rather than earlier in training.

Another new type of stress that you may encounter is that of, for the first time in your life, performing at an average, or even below average, level among your peers. As you well know, subtle details in verbal answers on the wards can often lead to harsh criticism and embarrassment. Additionally, if you haven't already been made to feel that you have not responded to some type of clinical demand fast enough, or been at the right place when you were needed, you most definitely will at some point.

If you are stressed out, this is completely normal. Medical training requires you to master a tremendous amount of information, the simplest of which is the notoriously high volume of memorization. Additionally, you must use your newly acquired knowledge to obtain clinical information from patients, and then make a decision regarding the patient's diagnosis and treatment. Then, you have to keep in mind potential side effects and alternative treatment options and make the right choice regarding treatment. In most cases there is no luxury of time to ruminate about your decision, as the patient will become sicker or clinically unstable.

And after you make your carefully thought out decision, you will be questioned by everyone involved in the patient's case, from other doctors, to staff, to the patient, the patient's family, and even the patient's friend, who saw a similar case on a TV show and thinks it should have been handled differently. There are multiple steps along the way that can lead to stress and anxiety.

The apprehension associated with criticism at this early stage is understandable and, unfortunately, standard. It is useful to keep in mind that the uncertainty of others around you can be masked as defensiveness among some of your peers, or even supervisors. However, while almost all doctors vividly recall too many medical school and residency days of enduring agonizing disapproval from senior residents and staff, most doctors have left the stress associated with their training long behind. Instead, practicing physicians hold on to the valuable patient care skills and professional discernment absorbed during the early years of training. It is not the clinical demands or difficult subject matter that causes practicing physicians to want to leave medical practice, but rather the systematic hurdles.

Tom Kelly, MD, residency program director at University of Chicago Department of Neurology says,

> I think the best way for coping with the stress of residency begins while still a medical student. The student should go into residency knowing this will be a stressful period in life, and not have any false illusions about that fact. In reality, before deciding upon a career in medicine, the difficulty of training should be taken into account. Once in training, I think the best approach

is to become efficient and knowledgeable in your field, and get the work done as soon as possible, and not let loose ends dangle. In addition to working hard and efficiently, one must strive for some balance in life, when possible, such as having interests outside the world of medicine. However these interests should not interfere with job performance. Yes, a resident is an employee as well as student, and it sometimes is an uncomfortable mix of responsibilities. I think the resident always sees the student aspect but forgets that residency is also a job, and learning this aspect of medicine will give perspective on their responsibilities and reduce stress, and prepare them for the "real" world, when, even as attending physician, they will be in subservient positions to employers and regulatory agencies. In short, realize stress is inherent to training, accept it, realize the training period is finite, make the best of it, learn all you can (even if from personal email exchange).

Dr. Kelly's comments summarize the two factors at play during medical school and residency very well. The training period itself has unique challenges that will only be present for a relatively brief period of time. However, the exposure to patient care as well as clinical practice regulations can demonstrate for a young physician whether the long-term environment of medical practice is indeed the right fit. Young physicians face the challenge of differentiating whether dissatisfaction is a symptom of the newness of medicine or of not wanting to be a doctor after finding out what it involves. The question may be—wait and see if I start to like it or get out now?

Unfairness

Sometimes the pressure and anxiety of medical training can be a result of factors that do not feel temporary, such as truly poor performance or unfair treatment. While it is not common, young doctors in training can experience real struggles related to racism, intolerance, and sexual harassment. All doctors, and in fact people in any profession may experience these issues, regardless of age. This is unfair, and it can be profoundly difficult to deal with, especially when one is not only young and inexperienced in the professional world, but also made to feel that just "being here" in the program is a privilege. In the medical world, due to the seriousness of outcomes, when a young resident is targeted as a "scapegoat," it can be overwhelming to deal with the consequences of this adult form of bullying, in combination with the regular challenges of training. Experience in the professional world can teach one how to manage such issues, but it is important for young physicians to understand that workplace injustice is not unique to your profession, or to your level of experience. It may be amplified due to your young age or lack of experience in the work environment, but it may occur for anyone because of the presence of poorly adjusted coworkers.

A doctor who had been new to the United States told me that she initially attempted to brush aside the issue of prejudice. Eventually, after she realized that it was not going to spontaneously end, she approached the subject with confidence by explaining the matter to an authoritative figure whom she respected in her training program. The problem was partially solved, but immaturity from fellow MDs regarding her foreign accent continued, while she rose above it. She values her experience, and has continued to promote an atmosphere of tolerance and patience in her current work.

I have spoken to many female physicians who have complained of sexism or harassment among colleagues and patients. Most have admitted that while it was frustrating, it was intimidating to complain about and difficult to define and express a substantial tangible consequence. But there is no doubt that uncomfortable situations in the workplace contribute to less than optimal performance, at the very least. Unfortunately, this reality is not only true in medicine, but in most fields as well—from the most highly qualified, to the most entry level positions. And witnessing discrimination of any type can affect your work, even when you are not the target.

Poor Performance

Although I addressed this subject in Chapter 1, it is so delicate a topic for most physicians that it deserves special attention in this section for physicians in training. While you are training, you are expected to be advancing and improving and learning. There are high expectations, and for good reason. The consequences of poor performance include less than stellar evaluations, as well as serious consequences for your patients. However, poor evaluations can provide an opportunity for targeted improvement in weak areas. There is a balance between the opportunity for improvement and serious penalties related to failure, being held back, or being removed from a program.

There is no "one size fits all" answer to poor performance. Practicing physicians who have been held back or failed at some point during medical school or training have been able to view the experience objectively and to get past it, mastering the material, without being subject to lingering consequences of early failures. Of the physicians I know who have done poorly in the past, all have remained in clinical medicine and are highly regarded as excellent physicians by patients, colleagues, and by themselves. Just as you learn to diagnose and treat patients' medical illnesses, you will have to learn to diagnose and treat any shortcomings that you demonstrate as a doctor.

But what if it is too late? What if you have been reprimanded? What if you have failed a licensing test or certification examination? What if you have lost your state license? It is completely beyond the scope and purposes of this book to advise you if you have done anything dishonest. But, if you made an honest error in some way—failed exams, poor judgment, clinical mistakes—you will need to do some soul searching and seek help. You cannot ignore these problems. You will have to familiarize yourself with the rules and regulations regarding your errors and the formal process for correcting them. You can determine which of the following—state medical society, state medical board, specialty society, specialty board, or hospital staff office—has the information and the step-by-step procedures that you need to properly correct errors.

You will need to approach this matter in a nondefensive way. One option could be to begin by writing out a formal request for rules and procedures. It makes sense to keep records of all action that you take to improve as well as all positive feedback that you receive. This will be helpful to keep you motivated, to remind you of your own improvement, and to objectively remind those evaluating you of your improvement in order to counteract any negative stereotypes or hearsay about you.

You should also turn to a trusted senior colleague in your field for advice. However, what if that is the person complaining about you? You can, and should, contact your former supervising doctors—whether they gave you good evaluations or not. How about those subpar evaluations from the past? Do they follow a common theme? Is there a way to fix this flaw? A few consistent flaws that a former residency program director shared with me that can cause repeated serious problems for physicians include: lack of knowledge, lack of confidence, stubborn attitude, defensive attitude, lazy, rushed, superficial, tends to blame others, temperamental, and distracted. Usually a doctor in trouble has the misfortune to possess more than one of these maladaptive traits. But they can be, and need to be, fixed. If it is too late for you to get back into medicine—even if you follow the rules—you should remember that you need to deal with these traits in order to avoid future problems and to be successful in your next endeavor, whatever it will be. Daniel Goleman's book *Social Intelligence* illustrates in a simple and straightforward way how habits of social communication can be deliberately enhanced and how these behaviors impact one's ability to function in a variety of situations. Another helpful resource for gaining better interactive habits at work is Tim Sander's *The Likeability Factor*, which simplifies the steps to gaining important practices of social interaction that can be lifesaving in the professional environment.

Missing Out

In addition to the stress that you find yourself having to adjust to at work, while you still have years of training and debt ahead of you, your peers in fields such as technology or business may boast that they earn more money than you, enjoy many perks, and have fewer work demands. This can lead young doctors in training to feel that they are missing out on life by spending a great deal of time studying and working in the hospital, while delaying the gratification of financial compensation.

A long-standing residency program director shares that this sense of uncertainty was particularly magnified for residents and medical students in the late 1990s, when an economic bubble formed in the United States, allowing many young college graduates to temporarily earn salaries much higher than they had ever dreamed of. Some of those young enthusiastic folks made wise decisions and managed their earnings quite well. Conversely, some were ill prepared for sudden layoffs or put their bubble-enhanced earnings into an inflated real estate market. The sad consequences for some have been dramatic, as those who believe in the fairy tale of a free lunch or a "new economy" tend to be the casualties of a harsh reality. While there is no crystal ball, level-headed decisions regarding finances will serve you well, whether you continue in a long career as a physician, or not.

One physician I spoke with was swept up by the popular day-trading trend about thirteen years ago. He took two years off from training and explored the world of day-trading hands-on. He describes his initial enthusiasm regarding his plan of leisurely days at home, studying the financial markets while wearing jeans and a sweatshirt, while his colleagues in residency spent nights in the emergency room evaluating chest pain. He explains that after a few months of intense anxiety spent following the stock market for the elusive purpose of making money, he wanted to get back into residency to work with real people. It took another year of waiting for a residency position to open before he could reenter the program. He says that he appreciates and values his medical education and life a great deal more after briefly "following his dream of financial independence."

If you feel that you may be missing out on other professional goals and opportunities unrelated to medicine, it is certainly worth your time to investigate and obtain accurate information about other fields that hold interest for you, rather than to wait passively. If you discover that another profession better suits you, there is no gain from remaining in a situation that is the wrong fit. I had the privilege of working as a neurologist in a well-established suburb of Chicago, Illinois. I saw a substantial number of migraine patients, and I learned from my patients that, behind the facade, the most stereotypically desirable jobs are often the source of many headaches—that cannot be treated by a neurologist.

Investigating professional alternatives thoroughly and carefully is a worthwhile investment of time, as mistakes can sometimes be costly and difficult to repair.

You should know that while most young doctors consider leaving medicine, most do not leave at this stage. And the majority of those who remain in the medical field find it satisfying. A marked advantage that midcareer physicians have is the mature understanding of the stresses associated with professional uncertainty in a variety of fields, not only in medicine.

Advantages for the Young Doctor

If you are a resident or medical student, you have the advantage of entering the medical field at a time when you and your contemporaries expect to have your eyes wide open. Your generation assumes that there is no reason to accept the structural limitations, or ambiguous regulations of any system. There is a better-balanced attitude in the physician's work environment, and cooperativeness among residents and an even-tempered demeanor is expected and supported in residency and medical school, which was not the case in the past.

At this stage in your medical career, it is less disruptive for you to make changes. You have better availability of resources within your medical school or hospital for participation in diverse medically related areas, such as healthcare economics, education, technology, or politics. This can allow you to explore your interests early on, so that you can decide whether you want to become more deeply involved in other aspects of medicine. You also have a better ability, at this stage in your career, to build your experience in these areas of focus. In addition, it is generally easier early in your training to reach out to mentors in your areas of interest and obtain internships and entry level positions, as you have the benefit of more direction and guidance from your training program now than you will have later.

You also have the advantage of entering the medical field at a time when your contemporaries have a markedly different attitude about the field of medicine. Adel Mahmoud, MD, Professor of Molecular Biology and Public Policy at Princeton University, observes that physician applicants to the highly competitive public policy program at Princeton range from faculty members to residents, and that they have the full encouragement of their programs in pursuing this degree. He states that it is a positive reflection of the current times that even prestigious surgery residency programs view the challenge and experience of a public health master's program as valuable for their residents.

The expectations that society and the medical field hold for future physicians will be forced to adjust to what the majority of young MDs consider acceptable. Newly trained doctors presume that they will be able to be engaged more actively in various aspects of healthcare, while maintaining the balanced lifestyle that they know is beneficial. Lorraine Millas of NeuroCall, Inc., a recruiting company for telemedicine physicians, states that the younger generation of doctors, while very dedicated to practicing good medicine, is not willing to give up a well-balanced lifestyle. She explains that both men and women physicians place an emphasis on time for family and a well-adjusted lifestyle and do not consider this attitude to be a stigma at all, as it was in the past.

A number of the physicians who shared their stories with me for this book pointed out the importance of an understanding of medical economics, finances, and policy for young doctors today. I personally recollect my days of training, and I do not recall that I had extra time to read books about coding, billing, or finances. However, as current doctors demand a well-rounded perspective for themselves, necessary education in practical subject matter such as healthcare finances may eventually become incorporated into medical education. It is certainly less frowned upon to express interest in understanding nonclinical aspects of medical practice during training. Even this small change is a great step in the right direction for future physicians as they manage their careers armed with better knowledge of the big picture.

Being a Good Doctor

Physicians in training and experienced doctors face many of the same motivating factors in considering the launch of a nontraditional career. The main difference lies in some of the details related to exit and in the available possibilities. The medical school I attended was a relatively nontraditional school, which took pride in the relatively high number of "bent arrow" students. These were students who had other careers prior to beginning medical school. A number of the students in my entering medical school class had been lawyers, accountants, engineers, and artists, and had decided to become MDs many years after finishing college. I recall a conversation between two first-year medical students—one was a youthful twenty-two-year-old and the other was a seasoned forty-year-old who had already had a career prior to entering medical school. The younger medical student asked the older medical student, "Do you know that in seven years you will be forty-seven years old, when you finally become licensed and can work as a doctor?" The older student answered, "I will be forty-seven in seven years whether I become a doctor or not. I might as well do something I really want to do."

In your case as well, you may not want to focus excessively on a perception of wasted years as you consider the possibility of changing your educational and career path at this stage. While medicine is known for being a profession for those who are capable of delaying gratification, you may be concerned that changing career paths will delay your gratification even more, to a degree that is intolerable.

While you evaluate your uncertainty about your career as a physician, you will undoubtedly contemplate whether you are more interested in becoming a skilled doctor, or in becoming something else. One of the difficulties associated with having doubts at an early stage is that you may be making a judgment about your long-term future while you are still experiencing a temporary stage that does not accurately represent the lifestyle, salary, or responsibility that you will live with as a practicing physician. It is critical for you to consider the question— do you want to overcome the stress of medical training in order to become a great doctor and take good care of your patients? Or do you just want to have a good job and make a lot of money? You should not continue to work at a job that is not the right fit for you if your goal is not unambiguously to become an outstanding doctor and take good care of your patients. This central point is important, because if you remain in medicine, your performance, your evaluations, and your professional reputation will be based primarily on your clinical proficiency, whether you choose a procedural or cognitive-based specialty. Your personal social skills will serve you well, but they will only complement, not replace, the requirement of first-rate clinical capabilities.

If your primary goal is something besides learning how to take excellent care of patients, you owe it to your patients, even more than to yourself, to get out of medicine. Your patients and their families deserve a doctor who cares about being a good doctor above other professional considerations. Whether you become a surgeon, critical care doctor, obstetrician, radiologist, or pathologist, you will need to methodically and carefully do your work well every time. You can make money doing other things if you do not enjoy the practice of medicine or do not want to excel at it. There is no doubt that if you were able to achieve well enough on your college classes and MCAT examination, overcoming the odds of entering medical school, that you can succeed in another field as long as you find it interesting, it suits your personal skills and abilities, and you apply your dedication to doing it well. You might find it helpful to review the professional criteria discussed in Chapter 4 as you evaluate your next step. There are so many nonclinical options for careers that truly help people, earn high salaries, or both. And, as you will see in Chapter 10, your medical training and skills will continue to serve you throughout your life in work and nonwork situations. You definitely have what it takes to succeed professionally, once you find the right fit for yourself.

3

Is It OK If I Leave Medicine?

One of the reasons that so many doctors who are drawn to alternative medical careers have not taken action is that there are some barriers to initiating a non-traditional path. It is because of these barriers that the decision to make a transition may not be simple or straightforward. The hurdles can be concrete and practical, such as financial constraints and scheduling matters, or more complex but nevertheless valid concerns, such as a sense of responsibility to patients or even qualms about social status. The key is to strive to gain perspective of the inhibiting factors in light of your long-term goals. The good news is that once these concerns are plainly understood and comprehensively addressed, they can be dealt with productively. See Figure 3.1.

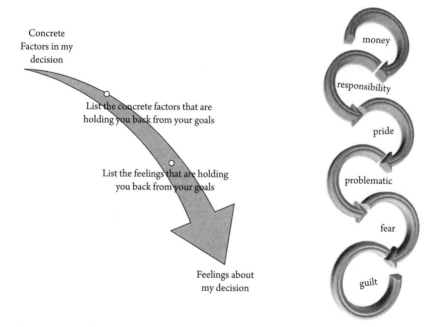

Figure 3.1 Can I leave medicine? The different factors at play.

It Has Already Cost So Much Money to Get Here

This is true and it can contribute a great deal to physician guilt in the setting of switching careers or slowing down. The financial cost, time commitment, and intense effort associated with obtaining a medical education are extremely high. Currently (and this number could continue to climb even higher) the cost of undergraduate tuition at a typical state university is approximately $20,000 per academic year. If you consider the expense of room and board, as is often necessary in order to attend college, the actual cost of attending a state university is approximately $40,000 per year. Medical school tuition ranges from approximately $30,000 per year to about $50,000 per year. Of course, living expenses, textbook fees, and travel costs for medical school visits and interviews, and, frequently, MCAT preparation classes, add to the financial burden. A very conservative estimate places a typical American medical school graduate with about $200,000 in educational expenses. So many doctors have told me that they asked themselves the question—could I leave medicine after I have paid so much money? What about all of those years of loan repayment? What if you aren't finished paying them back? This is definitely a valid point. Andrew Ibrahim, MD, who has written about cost issues in healthcare and medical education for various medical journals, including the *New England Journal of Medicine* and *JAMA*, effectively summarized one of the consequences of the high financial cost of medical education when I asked his opinion: "Physician debt can pigeonhole physician creativity, both within the medical field, and in preventing physicians from contributing to important issues, such as policy."

In addition to medical education, many physicians pay a fee in order to buy into a profit sharing partnership arrangement with an established practicing group. This cost is also a significant consideration for doctors who may want to transition out of clinical care prior to earning an income that may justify the entry fee into a group partnership. The variability of buy in and buy out or retirement details is vast and can work to the advantage or disadvantage of individual physicians who choose to leave the practice for any reason.

It is indeed realistic for you to expect the financial cost of your education, in addition to your time and hard work, to have an impact on your future earnings. However, you may have begun to consider that income is not the only factor that contributes to your professional happiness. Even if maintaining the equivalent of a practicing physician's income or higher is of considerable importance to you, many doctors I have spoken with about this subject emphasized that you should not consider your educational cost, time, and energy to be a waste if you pursue other options. If you leave clinical practice, you can certainly use your schooling, skills, and most importantly the confidence you gained after such challenging training to help you attain satisfaction based on your own criteria of professional and life success, including an income equivalent to that of a practicing physician.

Your medical background does not just boil down to tuition for lectures in physiology and anatomy. You are a doctor, and more than just a doctor, whether you practice clinical medicine or not. Physicians who practice medicine use their education and medical degree to help others directly in surgery, psychiatry, pediatrics, radiology, anesthesiology, and many more clinical specialties. Depending on your personality, your medical education, degree, and experience can serve as a background for a future career path that is right for you and that utilizes *both* your personal skills and your professional qualifications. Dr. Ibrahim, who is a painter, writer, and a physician, comments, "From my own experience, medicine is less of an end unto itself, but rather a platform to explore other areas of life. So the contributions of a physician to architecture, policy, painting...those are all underrated. We really should be balancing the increased specialization era we're in with more cross-discipline exchanges."

Jennifer Furin, MD, PhD, of the Department of International Health at Harvard University and Assistant Professor of Medicine and Anthropology, TB research Unit, Case Western Reserve University, encounters many doctors who think that they cannot follow their dream of international medicine work because of the balance of medical school loans. She says that there are many innovative programs for loan repayment such as Partners in Health, Project Blessing, and Catholic Relief and that resourcefulness and dedication are a great help in loan management. Physicians interested in pursuing public health and indigent care have resources that can assist them financially. Examples of resources for loan forgiveness include the National Health Service Corps, the National Institute of Health, the Indian Health Service, and rural health loan forgiveness programs, which often require specific types or locations of work as a condition for loan assistance. Similarly, Father David Milad, DO, who completed his residency in internal medicine prior to following his calling into the priesthood, says that there are select opportunities for physician clergy to apply for financial assistance with medical school loan repayment. Additionally, military loan repayment programs for medical school education generally require a specified duty to military service, and there are options for military physicians to do medical research or administration, not only clinical care. Most loan repayment and assistance programs tend to accept few applicants and are geared toward doctors entering professional arenas that utilize medical school education or postgraduate residency training in a service oriented manner or are associated with nonprofit work.

However, there are a number nonclinical work options, with a wide range of income levels. Maintaining a salary equivalent to or above that of a practicing physician can be a realistic target for physicians pursuing alternative professional opportunities, which can help in easing both the guilt and practical concerns regarding the expense of medical school education.

It Costs So Much Money to Leave

There is no doubt that medicine is not an easy career for transitions. Running a medical office requires a significant financial investment, and abruptly ending your practice will have a financial effect that extends beyond simply ending future income. If you modify your clinical practice, there are other expenses that you will need to continue to pay for some time to come. If you run your own medical office, you may need to continue to pay for your equipment costs, rent, and business support contracts such as billing services and electronic medical records payment and staff agreements even after you stop working. Self-employed physicians often have to accommodate their earnings pattern due to billing denials and long delays in payment for patient care services. As a consequence, while you have an ethical obligation to pay your staff and other overhead in a timely manner, your own revenue suffers great delays. Therefore, you may still have to pay your share in contracts extending beyond your own target date for leaving clinical work, while your collections will remain behind. If you are employed by a healthcare organization or by another physician, the biggest financial consideration is usually your malpractice tail cost, which is typically 2.5 times the cost of your yearly malpractice premium. Most physicians have an employment arrangement that features some characteristics of both self-employment and some characteristics of an employee. In many situations, the financial costs of leaving clinical practice, even to take a break, have been known to be prohibitive for physicians. If you run your own practice, you need to evaluate if it is possible for you to decrease your overhead costs, and possibly wind down, rather than suddenly close, your practice.

On a more positive note, most physicians have to deal with a few, but not all, of the above financial considerations when switching career paths. The exit costs as well as supplemental income options and their anticipated compensation are discussed in more detail in Chapters 5 and 6, as this can help ease the financial strain of leaving clinical practice. Because an MD can serve as a valuable instrument in the professional world, finding a good nonclinical job is not the limiting element for physicians stepping into alternative fields. Making a clean break financially is the most limiting factor for physicians who face this transition. In fact, I fear that the prohibitive cost of medical malpractice exit fees can effectively force physicians who should not even be practicing medicine to continue to practice.

While you obviously have to think about the practicality of the finances of your transition or exit from medicine, you cannot realistically force yourself to remain a captive to your initial decision to become a doctor if you are unhappy. This would be a disservice to your patients, and you may have other undeveloped talents that could be more beneficial for you, and for society as a whole. You can rest assured, however, that it is possible for you to map out a rational process for entry into another field, while maintaining an income that allows you to manage your educational costs and exit expenses.

I Have a Responsibility to My Colleagues

Before leaving, most doctors have considered the fact that they have a responsibility to their colleagues. While you and your colleagues would certainly be forced to rearrange your agenda on short notice if someone at work became sick, a purposeful transition in career goals may be viewed differently by colleagues. As with the financial matters discussed above, obligations to colleagues comprise concrete and practical facets as well as subjective components. Your fellow doctors have made call schedules, vacation plans, and a work routine that, in part, depend on you. Perhaps, as a solution, you can manage a modified work arrangement, such as cutting back on some clinical responsibilities while you continue to participate in patient care coverage on some weekends and holidays. A scheduling adjustment, in which you work out a fair compensation distribution, may be a logical approach for you and your partners. Be creative and sensitive with scheduling. Become aware of your physician colleagues' unique scheduling and work environment concerns, and contribute to easing these issues, so that you can remain a team player even on your way out.

It is typical to hesitate when it comes to sharing your plans with your fellow physician partners too far in advance. You would have a valid concern if you anticipate that your colleagues or supervisors would begin to look for another doctor to replace you before you are ready to leave. It is reasonable to be cautious, because your own transition timetable might not work out exactly as you would like. Therefore, it can be a tricky but nevertheless manageable process to conscientiously balance your contractual and ethical obligations to your work associates, with your own requirements for a degree of flexibility and some stability. You must appreciate that it is wise not to burn your bridges. You may continue to interact in some way with former colleagues even in your next nonclinical job. For example, you may end up starting a successful healthcare management company, and occasionally ask former colleagues to consult for you.

You have likely anticipated the need to prepare yourself for resentment, criticism, or even ridicule from other physicians. You may worry that other physicians could consider your decision to pursue a non-patient-care job be an indulgence. A physician who has been successful in the biotechnology industry agrees, "In some circles, talking about alternative careers would be looked down on. But do not give up on your ideas and plans because you are uneasy about losing status in the eyes of a few of your colleagues." You cannot please everyone—and you have worked far too hard to waste your time and energy trying to obtain approval from others. Your announcement may make some doctors uncomfortable, especially if they are already experiencing significant stress and conflicted feelings about their careers. However the only obligation that colleagues can ask of you is your fair and responsible transition, not a thorough justification of your change of heart.

Running Away

In the medical environment, there is often an attitude that only those who are tough enough get through. In the past, a number of residency-training programs were pyramidal, eliminating weak resident physicians each year. In fact, many demanding programs were known for scaring away fragile candidates from even applying. While this type of environment is less common in recent years, the attitude of sticking it out remains an integral part of the atmosphere of medical school, residency, and beyond. Doctors often have the outlook that leaving clinical medicine is fundamentally giving up on a difficult task. There is a tendency to view any deviation from clinical medicine as an acknowledgment of defeat.

Therefore, you may consider staying in medicine because you do not want to see yourself as the one who couldn't handle the pressure and ran away. And most doctors clearly remember at least one medical student or resident who had a meltdown and quit. In fact, most of us recall our colleagues discussing in whispers "what happened?" This typecast remains ingrained with so many doctors that over the years, it is presumed that whoever leaves just simply couldn't handle the pressure.

As mentioned earlier, running away will not achieve the outcome of making problems disappear anyway. If you have poor coping mechanisms, and most people have at least a few nagging imperfections, you need to tackle them eventually, whether you leave medicine or not. And you will only succeed in your next career phase if you proactively address these hurdles. You should not allow yourself to leave medicine in the context of running away, as this will leave you feeling that you have unfinished business in the long run. It makes sense to remind yourself of your valid motives for examining alternative jobs as you evaluate the basic career features that you desire in your work in the upcoming chapter. If you want to run away from medical practice, it is most likely not professional satisfaction that is binding you to medicine, but rather lack of an alternative plan. This does not mean that you would be incapable of handling clinical practice if you genuinely wanted to.

It Would Be Disruptive

This statement is accurate. There may be a degree of upheaval. And this, like the other factors listed above, can be a limiting factor if your current life situation is not receptive to disruption. However, most professionals, even physicians, have to deal with a degree of change in their professional lives at some time or another. MDs who remain in the medical field for their whole careers will eventually encounter modifications, such as associates relocating or retiring. Ambitious physicians may change jobs repeatedly, as they are frequently appointed to new leadership roles, sometimes requiring relocation to a new city. A good way to balance your concern about making too many changes with your aspiration to start a new career is to make a well-thought-out blueprint for your career change.

If you wish you could leave clinical medicine but you are more concerned about causing disruption, you should weigh whether your desire to leave medicine is stronger or your need for consistency. There is absolutely nothing wrong with staying in a job even when you know that there are other possibilities available to you as long as you continue to practice medicine with the high quality that your patients deserve. Your avoidance of disruption could essentially be an indication that your clinical practice provides you with more satisfaction than you realize. If this is your outlook, however, and concern about disruption is your main reason for not initiating an alternative career path, you should consider this a definitive decision to remain in medicine, not simply an acceptance of a bad situation. Many doctors have made positive career changes, and you have numerous options in medical practice and in different, nonclinical work. Consequently, having the privilege of being a doctor and acting disgruntled and trapped is not an option.

The Unknown

There is no question that medical practice follows a well-paved path and a relatively clearly defined work description. Often doctors who want to begin work in a nontraditional field do not know whom to ask about possible opportunities, because they may not know other doctors with relevant experience, in comparison to well-established patient care fields. There may be concerns about what to expect, including how to break into a nontraditional field, work environment, job security, job availability, and financial viability.

Emerging fields in the healthcare system are not well defined, and often the need for a new role is not fully grasped until after it is properly filled. Many doctors express frustration because they know that something should be done about the gaps in healthcare but that there is no existing entity or structure to get the job done. Therefore, clarifying the genuine need is often part of the challenge of beginning the path in a developing field. The medical environment is evolving in many ways. Improvements in technology often require a higher level of physician involvement. Increased patient access to and interest in healthcare raises patient expectations and heightens the need for better communication and education. If a doctor believes that healthcare is becoming more complicated, perhaps he or she would want to play a more active role in health care policy.

Doctors describe the outcome of extensively designed healthcare improvement overhauls as usually resulting in new checklists or requirements for healthcare professionals. This can result in a more fluid role for doctors with increasing informal responsibilities and functions that can overwhelm the traditional clinical obligations. This evolution of healthcare has carved out completely new physician functions without a well-established precedent. Typically, physicians, unlike other professionals, are not paid for the additional work of professional development and organizational management. Often, physicians have to take a new approach, defining a job as well as identifying approaches to pay for that position. Extra physician duties do not fit the current pay-for-service model of physician compensation. But payment models may have to adjust as the healthcare system continues to transform.

Katrina Firlik, MD, had been practicing as a neurosurgeon in a private practice group in Greenwich, Connecticut, with an academic appointment at Yale when she felt that, although her work was gratifying, she loves learning new things and wanted to start her own company. Dr. Firlik started by going to the technology transfer offices at local universities in New York City and Connecticut to get to know other entrepreneurs and what they were doing. She formed a network of people with interests similar to hers, but who had skills and experience that she did not have.

Her goal was getting patients to become more compliant with their medications. She says that as a neurosurgeon, she understood that it was difficult for patients to remember to take a medication to prevent stroke or heart attack ten years down the road. Dr. Firlik teamed up with someone who had experience in the gaming industry in Las Vegas, with a focus on understanding what makes people tick and rewarding patients for medical compliance with short-term rewards and incentives like points. She cofounded HealthPrize Technologies in September 2009. But who pays for this service? The pharmaceutical companies, who traditionally spend money in advertising to get new patients and doctors to start medications, have been recently shifting strategy in an effort to keep patients on their medications with medical adherence. Dr. Firlik's story demonstrates that new ideas without precedent or well-established value in the healthcare world can be effective and sustainable for physicians if they provide a needed service that has not yet been properly addressed. Doctors can succeed in unknown territory.

While this is can be a daunting challenge, it can also be an opportunity for using a medical education and experience to expand the spectrum of possibilities and make a positive impact on the world around us. Admittedly, in pursuing a nonclinical career, a physician often must tailor a self-directed educational path in addition to residency, often acquiring qualifications that are not as formally recognized as residency training but are nonetheless important. Your training and education can continue to be valuable as you search for another job. However, over time, your new work experience, in combination with your background as a doctor, will provide a clear picture of your value in your new role.

It Is Too Risky

Facing the unknown and following an uncommon or completely unique goal can be scary. While you might have a strong interest in a new career, or medical practice may be unpleasant for you at this time, medicine is what you are familiar with, and you know the rules. Admittedly, the rules for doctors sprout exponentially and may be becoming impossible for anyone to keep up with, but they are defined. New regulations certainly affect physician reimbursement, control of clinical decisions, and lifestyle for practicing physicians. Yet evolving rules may jumble or even eliminate the whole job description for some nonclinical positions. For instance, doctors who work in content writing for websites or blogs are subject to factors that are completely out of their control, such as changes in trends in communications and media or the fickle reputation of the web-based companies that employ them.

Yes, it is relatively risky to leave clinical medicine. While there are many jobs for doctors in a diverse array of alternative fields, in general, there is a greater possibility of job turnover than in medical practice. Ashraf Hanna, MD, PhD, vice president of commercial finance at Genentech, says that many small biotechnology firms may go out of business after only a few products fail. While having worked for one of these companies can serve as a background for finding another job in the growing biotechnology industry, there is less stability in most nonclinical fields than in clinical work. It is, however, subsequently easier to find a position in a nonclinical field after a framework of experience is established. Lewis B. Schwartz, MD, divisional vice president, Peripheral Drug-Device Combinations, Abbott Laboratories, says that jobs in the pharmaceutical industry often offer initial incentive packages upon hiring, which can ease the financial risk of taking a nontraditional job.

MDs in nonclinical work environments often must be more open to relocating than physicians in patient care practice. Some options, particularly in the entrepreneurial arena, are not suited for those with a low risk tolerance. However, a well thought out, rational plan, with solid backup options and a thoughtful provision for setbacks can lead to accomplishment of even uncertain goals for the right person.

Anthony Valenti, MD, cofounder and co-owner of a telemedicine company, offers an interesting perspective on risk. He says that start-up costs may be high when launching a business and that there is an inherent financial risk associated with leaving the well-established structure of clinical practice. However, he explains that the risk of medical errors and the risks of making a mistake with human lives outweighed the compromises with job security that he has made in his career. He says that any physician can recover from financial risk, thanks to the high level of education and skill set, but he explains that the consequence of a medical error is permanent for patients. Therefore, he believes that in running a company with a strong emphasis on minimizing medical mistakes, he has chosen an acceptable risk for himself, while reducing risk to his patients.

Inertia

This is a common reason for doctors to postpone the process of getting out of an unpleasant work environment or starting something new. Some doctors are so busy and consumed by their work that, even in a state of dissatisfaction, they wait for overhauls in their work environment to occur. Despite the constant progress in the field of medicine, the professional modifications that an individual doctor may need in order for the clinical practice to become more tolerable may not interest anyone besides that doctor. You may be dealing with an unsustainable situation in your clinical work setting, but if you remain unable to picture what you could do instead, or how to get there, you might, understandably, do nothing.

Inertia, like a fear of upheaval, is actually an indication that you either do not have a well-formulated plan of action or that, while you might complain about some aspects of your work as a doctor, you are generally satisfied. It is worthwhile to figure out if you need a spark to get moving or if you need to make your practice situation better for yourself. Continuing to make excuses such as, " I can't stand this job, but I don't know what else to do," serves no purpose, because there are alternatives.

A good way to overcome inertia is to begin by reading about your other field of interest. The Internet has made educating yourself about any subject remarkably easy (but also unreliable at times.) Investigation of various subjects of interest, such as healthcare technology or public health grants, can motivate you to get started in actively pursuing your goals. By creating a genuine picture of what you might do next, after evaluating your values and the available options, you will be more motivated to take action to realize your goals. It can be tough to make the transition, and formulating a plan using the steps outlined in the following chapters can help. However, if you decide that changing careers is too much trouble or will not satisfy you, then, as with fear of disruption, you must accept and embrace your career as a physician in order to better serve patients and yourself.

Family and Mentors

What about the sacrifices your family has made? If your family members helped you in paying some of your tuition and could benefit from your repayment to them, it would be fair to make a repayment schedule to allow them to live comfortably. If you are married, your husband or wife will be a partner in your career decision. If your spouse had to work to pay for your education and living expenses while possibly even sacrificing his or her own professional aspirations, clearly he or she will feel due for stability, financial security, and your professional satisfaction. Some physicians may feel that they are letting down mentors who advised them through the rigorous process of getting into and getting through medical school by teaching, writing letters of recommendations, making phone calls, and reviewing applications.

It is critical to acknowledge that your unhappiness itself cannot compensate those who have supported you during your education and training. But, at the same time, you already realize that you must fulfill your responsibilities to those who rely on you. Accordingly, in order to balance your aspirations with your obligations, it would be helpful to make a timetable in cooperation with those whose lives are directly affected by your plan.

Most people would agree that it is unfair to your family for you to abruptly quit working as a physician and begin going to art school if you have already purchased a house and a car that you can barely afford, causing your wife to suddenly have to look for a second job right after having baby number four. But, if a relative is going to be upset that she will have to stop bragging to her friends about the fact that you are a "doctor" you definitely deserve to give yourself a break on that one!

Doctors Help Sick People

The reality is, that very few jobs allow you to help people on a daily basis. And there is no debate that sick people need help. You know how to help them. You will be asked, "how could you waste your ability to help people?'" or "how could you take the privilege of being a doctor for granted?" After you begin talking about your possible exit from clinical medicine, you will certainly encounter someone who reminds you that you are capable of helping sick people and expresses to you that anything else you choose to do is inferior. And most surprisingly, the person who tells you this statement may not be another doctor. It will probably be a friend or acquaintance, who vividly recalls being deeply appreciative of a doctor. This is a valid point. You have the privilege of holding the knowledge and skill that is truly helpful to those in need. Many, many people you encounter will tell you that they wish they could help people the way you can. It will surely make you think twice.

Guilt about leaving patients and their difficult problems behind is a common reason for not taking a step that you want to take. It is normal to be concerned that if you leave medicine to do something else you may eventually feel that you have made a big mistake. It is important to clarify whether your hesitation about leaving patient care stems from guilt or from a sincere feeling that you will miss patient care. Your well thought out motivations are still there for you. How much time commitment and dedication you have decided to devote to your new field of choice, or to medicine, is really your decision and nobody else's. There are only twenty-four hours in a day. You will never lose the sensitivity and empathy that you have gained as a doctor. You just might apply those qualities to something else. You can begin by erasing the false value judgment that taking care of patients is better than nonclinical physician work. It is simply the prevailing structure with respect to physician training, not the only way that physicians can contribute to society.

Do I Have to Be the "Bad Guy"?

This question comes up often as well. The answer, contrary to popular belief, is "no." Many doctors view MDs who are employed in nonclinical work as contributing to the problem of administrative excess rather than helping streamline medical care. I worked as a physician reviewer for a major healthcare consulting company, while I continued to work as a clinical neurologist. I found that, while I was not happy with the fact that my own valid requests for brain MRIs were denied, my typical agitated response with the insurance company did not help the situation. When I tried to understand the reasons for the denials, I was able to change my own ordering process to become more efficient.

I eventually took a position working for that company. I found that I was able to develop relationships with our clients, the ordering physicians, and their staff, in order to better explain the process, and to make ordering imaging tests easier and more practical for the doctors and their patients. As a physician, working in a nonclinical setting does not necessarily require you to be the "bad guy." You have taken care of sick people. You know your values, and you know that you will not compromise them for the sake of producing pretty outcomes results on charts. I can undeniably say that I never compromised my principles of giving patients the best care they needed and I was never asked to.

Richard Smith, MD, MBA, a senior medical director at a leading healthcare management company, says that dealing with angry doctors is a part of the job in utilization review. I personally heard my fair share of physician philosophical input about the state of healthcare. In fact, a particular remark that I heard really stayed with me. One doctor told me, "Do you know how many people who have never laid eyes on this patient have had a say in her care?" As the medical system becomes more complicated, with regulations and mandates, physicians have to seize better opportunities, on many levels, to make the situation simpler, more practical, and effective, while improving the outcomes that matter most. See Figure 3.2.

Can I Come Back? Credibility

Many physicians recall early concerns about the viability of reentry into clinical practice after time off. They all shared the consensus that reentry into clinical

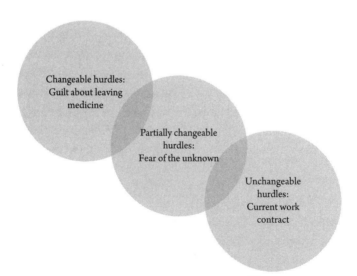

Figure 3.2 What is preventing you from doing what you want? List every hurdle that you consider important and put it in one of the three boxes. Then list the steps you need to make in order to tackle the hurdle.

practice remains an option for those who have left clinical work on good terms. Due to the high demand for physicians, clinical positions in just about every specialty remain unfilled, and a good qualified physician is always in demand. An interventional radiologist who took several years off completely from work when she had twins summarized her thoughts by stating, " I wish I knew that getting back into clinical practice is not as big of a deal as I thought it would be. I would have saved myself a lot of anxiety."

It is important to note, however, that licensing, recertification, and maintenance of certification, is becoming a more complicated, time-consuming, and expensive process in some specialties. April Confessore, a recruiter with Infinite Talent Medical Staffing, explains that physicians who take time off from clinical practice, for any reason, and want to come back, should preemptively prepare for simplifying the process of reentry by maintaining certification and licensure. Moreover, several specialties and states require continued clinical work in order to preserve specialty certification. In many such instances, nonprofit volunteering might serve to fulfill clinical requirements for certification while a doctor maintains full-time nonclinical employment.

There is a fine line between formal requirements and credibility when it comes to reentry into the medical field. The physicians with whom I spoke have echoed each other's comments that credibility is not as big a practical issue as it is a source of anxiety. Jennifer Furin, MD, PhD, who has worked on designing residency training programs for international health physicians at Harvard University, says that public health policy positions tend to be more appropriately filled by physicians who have already attained fieldwork experience and continue to remain in touch with the subtleties of patient care. This is a subjective opinion that may be shared by physicians in hiring roles for nontraditional jobs. In contrast, detailed requirements for certification and clinical practice may be mandated by companies in a number of nonclinical areas, such as in government agencies or in the healthcare insurance field, where a degree of continued clinical involvement and maintenance of professional licensure can protect a physician against changes in policy. Conversely, the pharmaceutical and biotechnology industries, which require scientific or business acumen, do not necessitate as much continued clinical involvement.

Conclusion: You Have So Much to Contribute

You, as a physician, have a great deal to contribute to the field of healthcare, even if you do not directly practice medicine. While only physicians with the medical degree and rigorous training that you received are permitted to treat patients, that fact does not mean that you are simultaneously limited to clinical

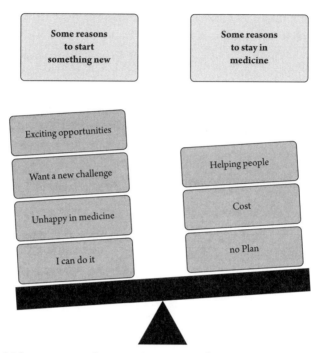

Figure 3.3 Make your own scale using YOUR reasons for wanting to start something new and your reasons for staying in medicine.

work. You have already seen patients as human beings, not profit numbers or "lives covered." Your involvement in healthcare policy, management, journalism, or administration provides value to patients and other healthcare professionals. You have so much to contribute. See Figure 3.3.

Healthcare is a rapidly evolving field. Patients expect to play a significant role in their healthcare decisions, increasing the need for patient education. Preventative medicine is helping people stay healthy longer, which intensifies demand for reliable public information. Advancing technology improves disease treatment, as well as healthcare delivery. Healthcare costs are an area of great controversy and misunderstanding. There is growing enthusiasm for correcting the disparities in healthcare, both locally as well as globally. With these changes, doctors are called on to do more for patients, in addition to patient care. Being a good doctor includes, but is not exclusive to, taking care of patients in the traditional clinical practice. With this transformation, new roles are created, and doctors often find that they must either find a balance or devote their time to new roles that do not fall into those of the traditional medical specialties.

As physicians, we have been able to see the success of our healthcare system and the real-life benefits that patients experience every day. Additionally, physicians and patients often criticize certain features of the state of healthcare. While

the problems in the healthcare system will not improve overnight, your frustration with some of the rules and ideas that interfere with good healthcare delivery
can translate into active participation in improving the system that you have been
a part of. You are uniquely suited and qualified to fill a much-needed gap in patient
care, healthcare delivery, or community issues if you want to do so. When doctors
approach problems in a substantial pro-active manner, they can truly alter the
world around them for the better. Whether you leave clinical medicine to teach,
become a hospital administrator, start a biotech company, serve in public office,
or run a music school, your genuine, balanced contribution to society as an intel-
ligent, caring doctor utilizing your medical background and nonmedical skills,
will serve to move medical care forward, not backward. You can continue to have
a positive impact, but in a different way than with patient care.

4

The Vision: What Do I Want to Do Next?

Once you have reached a clear understanding of why you want to initiate another career path and addressed the hurdles that may have been delaying your transition, you can begin to map out what you are going to do next. You are qualified for a wide range of exciting nonclinical work alternatives. You have so many choices, in fact, that you actually need to carefully and thoughtfully narrow down your selection in order for your job search and transition process to be efficient and effective. It is worthwhile in the long run to give yourself time, early on, to form a realistic image of the work that you truly visualize for yourself after you leave clinical medicine.

As you begin to put committed groundwork into your next steps, you can genuinely evaluate your personality along with your professional aspirations. Most doctors, whether they dedicate their entire careers to direct patient care or move into another field, are very ambitious. The style of ambition varies, however, depending on each individual. Your level of education, knowledge, skills, experience, and medical degree will continue to allow you to aim for financial security, a fulfilling job, a high-status position, meaningful impact on the world around you, flexibility, or a combination of any of these and other job attributes that you consider important.

Depending on a number of considerations, you may or may not place great emphasis on whether your career plan is one that can be economically reimbursed to your satisfaction. If you have decided to leave the field of medicine completely, so that you can dedicate your time to writing a memoir, for instance, you must have already concluded that you are in a financial position to give up your income. If you want to start a relief project for the underserved, you may be looking for ways to fund your project, and you might decide to continue clinical practice primarily to monetarily support your mission. On the other hand, if you are so dissatisfied with your job that you want to leave medicine but the only thing standing in your way is figuring out how to find an alternative career that pays reasonably well, potential income would be high on your list of priorities. Consequently, it makes a big difference whether your goal is to find another job to replace your medical practice or to cultivate a passion that you care about.

Because you have many parallel considerations to keep in mind as you make decisions that depend on one another and depend on a series of unknowns, a straightforward stepwise progression may not always be possible. If you want to lead a statewide program to improve prenatal care for teenagers, for instance, you might estimate that you will need to cut back your practice by two days a week. In the meantime, you may need to discuss with your physician partners the financial implications that such a change would have on your group practice. But you could be hesitant to start making plans to cut back on clinical work because you are still waiting for funding for your project. To complicate matters even more, you might not be ready to commit to relocation for your new venture because of ambiguous obligations with your current practice. As you systematically proceed with your transition, you will get the answers to your many questions, and that will help you to decide on your next steps.

Narrowing Down Your Choices

If you have not yet selected specifically what type of job you want to look for, you are certainly in good company. There are many alternatives for MDs seeking nonclinical work. However, physicians often discover at this stage that searching for "nonclinical jobs for doctors" or "medical field jobs" yields nonspecific results rather than real job opportunities. There is no job with the title Non-Clinical-Doctor. Similarly, there is no job description for "a doctor needed to do important work, no patient care duties."

Hence, searching for a career without a specific job title or description will ultimately lead to frustration rather than to measurable progress. Moreover, if you proceed to inquire about an eclectic assortment of nontraditional job prospects, you could end up unnecessarily wasting your valuable time on your job quest and transition process. The breadth of your efforts can interfere with the depth, which may result in a lack of focus. This can ultimately reflect on the quality of your contact correspondences, CV, and interviews, and prevent you from demonstrating that you are as qualified and prepared as you really are.

A university department chairman of a behavioral health department recollects interviewing a physician who seemed apathetic and even generic in an interview. The department chairman explains that his impression of the MD was that she was looking for any escape from medicine, rather than truly motivated to contribute to his department in a meaningful way. Lewis Schwartz, MD, also observes that many doctors know that they do not want to see patients but are not sure what they want to do. This can result in physicians being directionless even after acquiring a nonclinical position.

Doing Your Homework

You have the opportunity to evaluate your impression of numerous work opportunities for doctors in Chapter 5. A number of your options in alternative medical arenas may appear interesting to you. And, given your high qualifications, you are likely to get job offers in several of the fields described, with a reasonable amount of effort and determination. However, as I will discuss in Chapter 7, your application and interview process will be meaningfully more effective and will yield the best results for you, if you put your time and energy into logically researching your specific industry of choice. This will provide you with a no-nonsense understanding of the work expectations and the environment of the companies and organizations that you wish to work with. You will gain an advantage of approaching meetings and interviews in a confident, realistic, and well-informed manner.

As you already know, which of the many opportunities that you ultimately choose to concentrate on will depend in large part on your priorities. Tightening your search at this time will improve your likelihood of finding and succeeding at your next job. Therefore, you should first identify the fields, and types of jobs that will be professionally fulfilling for you.

The Differential Diagnosis

As discussed in Chapter 1, you might not have a specific job in mind. Instead you may have a need to leave medicine, or even an appetite for a different work environment, or a vague sense of dissatisfaction. That is not unusual, and will not limit you from finding a rewarding career path. If you have not chosen to pursue another specific job, it is well worth your time to begin by identifying your priorities. You have professional and personal ambitions that were at least partially fulfilled by your decision to enter the medical field. After you worked for some time in medicine, you may have realized that some of the goals that you consider important are not being attained in your medical job. It is not unusual to acquire new goals during your professional life. Several doctors I spoke with echoed each other's reflection that the decision to enter the medical field is often made at a young age and that priorities often change over time.

It is critical at this point to carefully capture the *elements* of work and life that are important to you. This will allow you to find a custom fit for your next step, including the ideal combination of clinical practice with your nonclinical interest.

Some of these elements are concrete, such as time, money, and location, while others are more intangible, such as a drive to serve others. You are a physician with advanced training and experience, confidence in your ability to achieve academic success, and a relatively high earning potential. The years, financial cost, and energy that you have already expended in order to attain your position as a doctor are traditionally viewed as a prerequisite to earning a high income. But for many, a greater value is placed on professional components like job flexibility, being one's own boss, or being in a position to take initiative. Your choices will reflect your own values. There are alternatives for you that incorporate your values. The following professional and personal priorities are specifically examined in light of your background as a physician. Even if you have decided that you want to commence a specific non-patient-care career, an evaluation of your priorities at this time will help you decide if the career you have in mind is actually in line with your goals.

Time

- How do you want to allocate your time?
- Do you want to leave medicine because you are dissatisfied with the time demands?
- Do you want to divide your time between medicine and another project or career?
- Which activities are important to you?
- Is time for family, recreation, hobbies, or leisure important to you?

Before you begin to pursue another job, you should honestly assess your level of anticipated time commitment to your next job. Additionally, you have to evaluate whether the time that you are willing to devote to your endeavor can serve to provide you with your aspired income level.

Money

- Is money a major motivating factor for you?
- Do you view money as a measure of self-worth, security, status, or a means for enjoyment?
- How much could you tolerate a drop in income?
- Are you driven to leave medicine primarily by a desire to increase your salary?
- Can you tolerate financial risk?
  Do you view your income as enough? More than enough? Not enough? Why?

- And equally important—how about your family, and the people who depend on you to support them? Are they willing and able to tolerate a change in your finances?
- Have you thought about employment benefits?
- How does your future estimated income fit into your plans for investment and retirement?
- Are you secure financially, or do you maintain a reliable income from other investments so that income is not a major factor?
- Do you need to secure funding for your next endeavor? Do you know how to obtain funding, or do you want to learn how?

Money is a basic necessity in life, yet also has meaning for individuals that can be very complicated. On a basic level, maintaining an income to preserve or improve a consistent standard of living, and to avoid financial stress, is important for most physicians, except for those who had been prepared to retire from work. It is important to comprehensively address all financial issues and map out a thorough monetary transition plan in order to make sure that the concrete aspects are addressed ahead of time. Tools for calculating budget questions are provided in Chapter 6. Some physicians might consult a financial advisor if the financial planning is particularly complex. However, for some, deeper considerations related to income, such as the perceptions of others, may play a disproportionate role in decisions related to work and spending. It is critical for individual physicians to understand their own views of money, and to properly address any knotty issues that may cause flawed decision-making before proceeding with a career change.

Social Status

- How important to you is the social and society prestige associated with being a doctor?
- Will you remain satisfied with your new job or position if you give up that social status?
- Do you feel appreciated by patients and coworkers because you are an MD? Do you think that you will have less esteem for yourself if others do not identify you as a doctor?
- Do you hold or show greater or less value and respect for family members, friends, or coworkers who are not doctors? Why?
- Are the people in your life who are important to you also doctors? Will you lose some of those connections if you leave clinical medicine?

- Have you allowed another person's definition of value to cause you to remain in a job that you do not like? More importantly, can you, and do you want to, change your definition of self-worth to include your other characteristics besides the fact that you are a physician?

The previous questions are often uncomfortable for physicians to discuss openly, but at least giving them private thoughtful consideration yourself can help you understand some personal factors that may play a role in your decisions. If you decide that you want to transition into another field but that you have a strong need to be addressed as "doctor" either socially or professionally, while you will need to exclude some potential options, you still have many professional nonclinical alternatives.

Professional Status

- How important is it to you to be highly recognized in the work setting?
- How much do you care about what people see when they search you on the Internet?

For many professionals, the recognition attained by work achievements is very important. In most medical careers, acknowledgment and appreciation is a daily occurrence yet is individual in nature. In this modern time of the Internet, when many people are more publicly recognized than in the past, some physicians may prefer to attain professional status on a wide-scale level for many reasons, including building a more reputable CV.

Medical Background

- Would you be happy in a position that does not require or value your medical expertise?
- Are you preoccupied with the idea that you may have wasted your education and training if you do something besides patient care?

If you decide to invest time or expense in the pursuit of another professional career path—such as business, real estate, law, education, or technology—will you expect to continue to incorporate your medical background in your future work? As you already know, if you obtain another degree, you might be able to market yourself as a businessperson specialized in heath-related investments, a lawyer working for health regulators, or a biotechnology specialist. It would be beneficial, before you commit yourself to a lengthy and costly educational program, to decide whether you truly want to incorporate your medical background into your future—or whether you feel obligated to. This can help you to decide which direction is most suitable for you.

Location

- Do you want to stay in your community?
- Would you be willing to relocate if an alternative work opportunity became available in another city or state?
- On the other hand, is the possibility of moving to a different community an attractive part of your plan?
- Are you in a position that involves travel for lectures and CME? Can you give up that perk? Or do you consider your current level of work-related travel to be a burden?
- Would you be willing to travel more frequently for your job? Does the prospect of increasing or decreasing your work or leisure travel play a role in your motivation for pursuing another professional interest?

Michael Lombardo, MD, a physician executive at a large hospital system explains that because of a slow housing market, he was unable to sell his home in a small town in Pennsylvania, and therefore commuted to another state for several years, eventually selling his home at a loss in order to move his whole family closer to his work. Prioritizing whether you care more about location, or about the timing of your transition may become a factor in evaluating some nontraditional opportunities, and can determine, to an extent, whether or not you have many or limited options in your job search.

Learning Something New

- Do you have a nonmedical personal or professional interest that you would like to pursue further?
- Are you interested in developing new skills and obtaining new knowledge?
- Are you looking for new professional challenges?
- Do you have personal or professional strengths that you wish to further develop? For example, are you a good teacher who wishes you could devote more time to teaching?
- Do you have specific gaps in your skills or knowledge base that you would like to allocate more of your time to improving? For instance, are you lacking in business

skills yet finding that you do not have the time to advance your understanding of this subject with your current work demands?

- Are you committed to learning about a particular topic of interest to you? Are you interested in formal instruction to learn about your interest or to better develop strengths? It has been fascinating for me to hear from several physicians who have been willing to pay for formal instruction and courses in diverse subject matter, such as computer skills or nutrition, which may not directly lead to any income.
- Have you been waiting to develop a particular talent of yours that has not been satisfactorily utilized in your current work, such as public speaking, writing, or mentoring?

Adel Mahmoud, MD, Professor of Health Policy at Princeton University says that he was drawn to his previous position as chairman of vaccines at Merck Pharmaceuticals because he thrived on the opportunity to learn something new, and wanted the opportunity to approach medicine from a different angle. Dr. Mahmoud has had a varied career in medicine, achieving a high level of success in each different setting. He was chairman of internal medicine at Case Western Reserve University for twelve years, and a well-known authority on tropical medicine, when he was approached by Merck Pharmaceuticals to become president of Merck vaccines. He states that he accepted the position because, he admits, that he cannot put up with too steady of a life and that he is always looking for new challenges and fresh ways of thinking. And, at Merck, he says, he welcomed the task of starting over with a new approach to medicine, almost from scratch, absorbing and learning as much in his first year in the pharmaceutical industry as a fresh postdoctorate fellow.

After retirement from a successful tenure at Merck, instead of pursuing familiar territory and taking another clinical department chairmanship or medical school administrative role, he chose, instead, to pursue yet another completely new role, as a Professor of Undergraduate Biology and Public Policy at Princeton University. He says that he had never taught undergraduate students before his position at Princeton, and that undergraduate teaching offers completely different challenges and is more deeply involved, in many ways, than teaching at the medical school level.

Dr. Mahmoud's story illustrates what many in the healthcare field have observed—that physicians with a well-established track record are often sought out by industry as leaders. He changed gears several times and was able to continue to learn new things. But the reason that he was recruited as a newcomer to industry and then, later, health policy education was because he had so much to contribute to each new niche of medicine based on expertise from the previous area. He accepted and welcomed these transitions because he considers new environments and approaches to be exciting and challenging.

Learning something new can be a type of benefit of a job in and of itself, more valuable than payment and worth paying for for many doctors.

Who Is the Boss?

- Are you intent on carving out a work setting that will allow you to take more responsibility for your productiveness and to be your own boss? How do you feel about the prospect of managing many employees? While autonomy can be liberating and challenging, it can also lead to demanding work obligations.
- Do you prefer a job that does not involve responsibility for employees or for the company's overall performance? Do you favor working as an employee?
- Would you find freedom in a career path that allows you to take time off without having to think about work?

Regardless or your job setting, you will have a boss. Do you prefer to work for an individual, a large system, or yourself? An experienced, self-employed family doctor once told me, "I have hundreds of bosses. Every patient and every patient's family is my boss."

Don't Repeat the Past

- Are you fed up with certain aspects of your job and leaving medicine primarily to avoid specific aggravations as discussed in Chapter 1?
- Is your motivation for changing jobs prompted by your intention to avoid irritating or even intensely stressful aspects of medical work?

It would be helpful to be aware of what pushes your buttons as you gauge your many options. Different types of stress are more tolerable for different people. Within clinical medicine itself, trauma surgeons master the emergent stress of making life and death decisions at a moment's notice, while psychiatrists perform their jobs by listening to patients relive agonizing emotionally traumatic events. Many doctors who are not in either of these two fields may find the daily work involved to be too nerve-racking. Similarly, in the nonclinical setting there are different types of stress that may be tolerable, even enjoyable for some doctors, and irritating beyond measure for others. Some may enjoy supervising employees, while others may be excited by the challenge of meeting numerical business goals. Conversely, those tasks could be seen as miserable daily work for others.

Your Definition of Boundaries

- Do you feel that work and life should be separate?
- Do you feel comfortable taking care of work responsibilities at home and/or home tasks at work?
- Do you expect complete dedication from your coworkers while at work?
- Do you or your family consider your job to be intrusive to family life?

Your individual personality and preferences play a large role in what type of work situation could make you happy, productive, and successful. Some people have a strong preference for compartmentalizing various areas of their life. For example, some physicians enjoy the high-paced work of emergency medicine, and value the fact that this job allows them to return home after a long day's work and effectively "turn off" their pagers.

Other doctors, on the other hand, have a strong appreciation for the benefits of computer systems that allow them to look up patient laboratory and imaging results from home, hours after leaving the hospital or office. The ability to remain connected with work while at home and to continue to manage ongoing patient care issues is highly valuable to many physicians. Similarly, when you are determining which nonclinical field to pursue, you should keep in mind how separate or connected you would like to keep your work from your life.

Work Environment

- Do you like working in a group setting?
- Do you like making collaborative decisions?
- Do you appreciate or resent input from others?
- Do you like to see immediate results, or do you prefer long-term projects?
- Do you consider meetings to be a distraction from work or a valuable part of your job?
- Do you prefer a structured routine at work?
- Do you thrive on a variety of challenges in your work?
- Is it very important for you to be in a pleasant work environment?
- Do you enjoy mentoring others?

You might like working on a team, using feedback and building on other's ideas, or you may prefer to work on your own without having to take responsibility for coworkers' shortcomings. It is useful to consider whether you are adept and sensitive at the skill of training those who may be less experienced than you are. You could consider whether you need to attain a sense of accomplishment frequently on many tasks or less frequently on large projects.

Professional Blueprint

- Do you aspire to become an expert in a field?
- Do you consider academic knowledge and expertise a worthwhile goal?
- Or do you consider refining a specialized skill to be most valuable?
- Are you particularly interested in leadership positions? Do you want to be a leader so that you can gain the ability to get things done and have an impact?
- Do you seek to obtain a specific title or rank?
- Do you value stability or advancement in your professional life?
- What contributes to your sense of achievement?
- Are you interested in business?
- Do you consider changing your professional route to be an exciting possibility, or a sign of immaturity or flakiness?

In the book *Strategic Career Management for the 21st Century Physician*, the author, Gigi Hirsch, MD, highlights four basic career concepts. The linear career view revolves around climbing the ladder in a hierarchy. The expert view relies on improving technical expertise. The spiral concept is defined by broadening knowledge in a manner that requires previously acquired skills to open the door to new opportunities and skills. The transitory path follows novelty and new experiences and places less emphasis on using previously acquired skills. These four concepts may help you define which career path you would be most interested in following in your transition to a nontraditional career.

Serving Others

- Have you developed a passion for a specific cause or disease that you treat as a physician? Are you looking to devote more professional time to the treatment, research, or policy relating to a specific medical condition?
- Do you have a drive to solve a specific problem?

- Are you interested in social or political activism? Has your medical work made you aware of a social problem that lacks adequate solutions?
- Are you interested in working with individuals one by one or in having an impact on large groups?
- Do you consider the local or the global implications of your work to be more important?

Most doctors take some time to consider the particularly relevant question of how important it is to be able to help others. You have been training or working as a doctor, and the most basic definition of what you do is "helping sick people." If you want to leave medicine, in contrast to being drawn toward another field, how will you feel about working in a field that does not directly help people the way medicine does? As discussed in Chapter 2, many physicians and even nonphysicians consider the work of helping sick patients more satisfying and important than any other work in the world. If you embrace that value system yourself, do you feel that you need to transition into a profession that allows you to continue to directly help others?

Judy Willis, MD, MEd, was a busy practicing neurologist. She noticed, as a neurologist, that many of her pediatric neurology patients were not taught to their optimal learning potential, and that their parents did not have the tools to address that problem. She felt motivated, after fifteen years of clinical practice, to use her neurological expertise to address learning strategies. She left clinical practice and obtained a master's degree in education. Using the combination of her practical experience with pediatric patients, her neurological knowledge, and her educational degree, she has written numerous books about education and gives presentations and workshops to educators and parents, both nationally and internationally, about how the brain learns. Her teaching experience has ranged from elementary and middle school to undergraduate and graduate level teaching. She currently teaches as adjunct faculty at the University of California, Santa Barbara, and spends much of her time traveling as a speaker.

Dr. Willis, like so many physicians, noticed issues that are not directly regarded as the realm of doctors. While it is often an uphill hike without a clear map, there are benefits to society when there is such interplay between medical expertise, and problems that are not traditionally addressed by the physicians. Dr. Willis's overall job is not one for which there is a simple job description—medical education learning expert, author, and speaker. In situations like this one, when a doctor carves out a new function, the value may not be fully appreciated until some time after the new role is created.

Patience

- Do you want to get out of medicine as soon as possible?
- Are you waiting to find the perfect fit in your next job?
- Are you willing to dedicate a good deal of time and effort now to look for a new job?
- Are you interested in finding alternative work, but prefer to take a more leisurely approach to your job search?

This has a great deal to with how much you want or need to leave medical practice. It will take some time and dedication to find a new job. The more particular you are about the necessary features that your next job will entail, the more difficult it will be to fulfill these criteria. You can find a good alternative within a reasonable amount of time if you are dedicated to a job search and if your timetable is short. If you are looking for a dream job, however, or if you are not interested in making a dedicated effort to the job search process, it may take you longer to fulfill your criteria.

Evaluating Your Criteria

These are all important questions that you can use to help yourself visualize what you would like to pursue and to decide if a particular job could really fill the criteria that you need to be happier than you are now. After carefully considering the questions above, you will have a reference with which to approach the following list of professional priorities that apply to physicians. It would be useful to evaluate the criteria below and to assign 1/3 of the features listed as very important to you, 1/3 as moderately important, and 1/3 as unimportant. Whether you are frustrated or satisfied with medicine, whether you think that you have made a mistake in entering the field of medicine or not, you should begin the next professional step with an authentic awareness of your priorities and how you will proceed to achieve them. After rating these priorities, see the chart of alternative careers for doctors to see which priorities are satisfied by alternative careers (Table 4.1).

- Time
- Money
- Social status/Recognition
- Financial security
- Job security
- Job availability

Table 4.1
Chart
1 = minor characteristic
2 = medium characteristic
3 = major characteristic

	Money	Time	Patience	Social Status	Financial Security	Job Security	Job availability	Working Independently	Working on a team
Patient Care	2	3	1	3	2	3	3	2	2
Academic Research	2	3	3	3	3	2	2	2	3
Industry Research	3	2	2	1	3	1	3	1	3
Laboratory Work	3	2	2	1	2	2	3	3	1
Hospital Administration	3	2	3	3	2	1	1	1	3
Disability/Long Term Care	2	2	2	1	2	2	2	3	1
Insurance Work	3	2	2	1	3	2	3	2	3
Business	3	2	2	1	2	1	3	1	3
Technology	2	2	2	1	2	1	2	2	2
Teaching	1	1	2	2	2	3	2	2	2
Public Education	1	1	3	2	1	1	1	2	1
Writing	1	1	3	1	1	1	1	3	1
Regulatory Oversight	1	1	2	1	2	2	2	2	2
Risk Management	1	1	2	1	1	1	1	1	3
Public Health	1	2	3	2	2	1	1	1	3
Policy	1	2	3	2	2	1	1	1	3
Entrepreneurial	3	3	3	2	1	1	1	2	2
International Health	1	2	2	3	1	1	1	1	3

	Being your own boss	Heavy Responsibility	Creativity	Teaching	Learning	Autonomy	Entrepreneurship	Passion for a cause	Serving
Patient Care	1	3	2	2	3	1	2	3	3
Academic Research	2	2	3	3	3	2	1	3	2
Industry Research	2	1	2	1	3	2	1	1	1
Laboratory Work	3	2	1	1	1	2	3	1	1
Hospital Administration	2	3	3	2	3	2	1	2	2
Disability/Long Term Care	2	2	1	1	1	2	1	1	2
Insurance Work	1	2	1	1	2	2	1	1	1
Business	1	2	2	1	2	2	2	1	1
Technology	1	1	2	2	2	2	2	1	1
Teaching	2	1	3	3	2	3	1	2	1
Public Education	3	1	3	3	2	3	2	2	3
Writing	3	1	3	3	2	3	2	1	2
Regulatory Oversight	1	2	1	1	2	2	1	1	2
Risk Management	1	1	1	3	1	2	1	1	1
Public Health	2	3	3	2	3	2	2	3	3
Policy	1	3	2	2	3	2	1	2	2
Entrepreneurial	3	3	3	1	3	3	3	3	2
International Health	2	3	3	3	3	2	1	3	3

- Working independently
- Working on a team
- Being your own boss
- Level of responsibility
- Teaching
- Learning
- Making the rules vs. following rules/Autonomy
- Entrepreneurship
- Creativity
- Passion for a cause
- Serving an underserved population
- Patience

Your views of these priorities may have been surprising to you if you have not thought about some of these questions recently. Additionally, due to your own unique situation, you probably have other job criteria that you are searching for, and you will undoubtedly keep those in mind as well. As I discuss very specific potential nonclinical opportunities and their characteristics in the upcoming chapters, you will see how some nontraditional medical careers could serve to fulfill your criteria and expectations more than others. If your vision of the future did not clearly delineate a specific dream job, you can now implement your specific dream job *criteria* to actual jobs.

With a realistic image in mind, you will be better able to begin investigating potential opportunities. It is helpful to think about how you picture your future prior to the initiation of your job search. You can and should begin to make choices about what you envision as a typical work day or work week in your next career; what you hope to accomplish over the course of the next year, five years, and ten years; and what type of lifestyle you expect to attain. This will help you to eliminate opportunities that do not match your goals.

Once you begin to form a picture of what you want in the next professional stage of your career, you will also need to prepare yourself to allow for the flexibility to make changes to your plan as necessary. As you begin to make progress in your quest for your next job, you will be pleasantly surprised with career scenarios that you had not directly been looking for.

Just a Small Change

It is worth noting that, as you think about your ideal job features and your goals, that you may decide that you would prefer to switch to another clinical practice arrangement or medical specialty, rather than entirely leaving clinical medicine. You can examine many of the nontraditional clinical work opportunities in Chapter 5. But traditional medical practice itself offers such a wide variety of work situations that it would be negligent not to mention the expansive variety of options.

A doctor can work in private practice, either solo or with a group, taking significant accountability for reimbursement and business decisions in addition to the responsibility of the medical care of patients. A physician can work as staff doctor in a hospital, medical institution, or managed care organization, taking responsibility for patient care and documentation related to patient care and billing but avoiding contractual deals related to the organization. Additionally, MDs can take positions that include a component of education and interaction with medical students and residents or not. Doctors can practice in settings serving working-class, affluent, or uninsured patients of any age, in an urban, suburban, or rural setting in any city or state.

Medical specialties offer a wide scope of work environments as well. As a pathologist, a physician spends a great deal of time identifying and interpreting the features of tissue specimens, most often in an academic setting. As a surgeon, a doctor uses technical skills along with clinical decision-making skills to directly treat patients. As a primary care doctor, a physician has long-term care responsibility for patients as well as health maintenance. As an emergency medicine physician, a doctor can take care of urgent medical needs and literally "save lives" on a regular basis. And as medical specialists, such as oncologists, pulmonologists, neurologists, or rheumatologists, physicians can become experts in complex fields, offering their patients updated knowledge and treatment. While this is only a brief summary of a few of the variations within the medical field, it is a crucial reminder that clinical medicine itself offers diverse opportunities. Even those who want to do something else may find it satisfying to make a modification in medical specialty, or even to simply change the type of medical practice setting within the same specialty.

The Plan

With these considerations in mind: the work criteria discussed above that you have selected as valuable, your relative interest and your ideal combination of your current and future field, and your ideal timetable, you can now seriously consider and map out your transition agenda.

As you chart out your best transition schedule, you will also have to consider whether you need a backup plan. Of course, your next job will not be perfect. The cliché is true, and the grass is not always greener on the other side of the fence. You could choose to change gears completely and, for example, open your own restaurant. You may look forward to the idea of finally serving people in times when they are in a good mood, in contrast to when they are sick or agitated and without the element of a third-party payer. However, you should keep in mind that you would be trading in one set of professional stressors for another. You will continue to have responsibilities, irate customers, and financial demands.

Because you probably have high ambitions, it is critical to reflect on the fact that your next endeavor will provide you with the prospect of professional satisfaction but also with new challenges. It is wise to anticipate that, regardless of your nonclinical choice, you will choose a professional path with inevitable negative features. Therefore you should undertake only those negative features that you consider acceptable and manageable.

When you consider the practical matters, such as which of the fields described in Chapter 5 suit your goals, how much you can expect to earn in Chapter 6, and how to proceed with the process of finding a job in Chapter 7, you can then adjust your ideal schedule to fit your practical, realistic, manageable timetable with step-by-step goals. A month-by-month job search and transition schedule will help you to see your goals clearly. After you read Chapter 7, you can then break down that schedule into a more detailed week-by-week schedule. This will include the detailed plans regarding researching job prospects, adjusting your CV and cover letter, making contacts, follow-up, and interview scheduling.

Your likelihood of reaching your objectives depends on your realistic understanding of your future field, and your level of dedication. As you continue to read valuable and honest advice from doctors who have achieved success in nonclinical medicine in the following chapters, you will gain an understanding of the expectations and anticipated environment of your next phase of professional development.

SECTION TWO

THE FACTS

| 5 |

What Else Am I Going to Do Anyways?

A World of Opportunities

If you have already established a definite career goal for the next professional chapter of your life, your energy will be focused on securing a position in your new, nonclinical setting. However, you may want to leave clinical work, but you might not know what else is out there for you. At this point, you have spent years absorbed in premed classes, MCAT preparation, medical school studies, and long residency nights on call. If you want to conclude your clinical practice, but have accumulated educational debt, or face the prospect of a medical malpractice tail fee, while you have not made any progress in becoming more qualified for another field, you may wonder if your only option is to continue the conventional practice of medicine. Your medical school preparation and guidance was geared toward residency and traditional medical career paths. You have been, like other physicians who wish to leave clinical medicine, unable to find reputable information and direction about how to enter the world of nonclinical medicine.

The fact is that you are more prepared for your next career phase than you may realize. You have medical expertise and possibly even specialty proficiency as well. You have worked directly in healthcare, which has exposed you to people of different backgrounds in their time of need. You have seen firsthand the many accomplishments of our healthcare system, and you have had to deal with the shortcomings as well. This background, in combination with your own unique personal abilities, positions you to make an effective transition into a new job that suits your professional skills and needs.

The following job options utilize your experience so that you can take advantage of your background. Many of these positions can be combined with clinical medicine or can serve as full-time employment. Some of the following options also offer the opportunity to supplement your income during your transition to a more long-term career. See Table 5.1.

Table 5.1 **Alternative Job Options for Doctors**

Scientific Research Jobs
University
Health Care Manufacturing Industry (pharmaceutical, product development)
Government Agency
Private Scientific Research Company
Medical Lab Opportunities
Owner
Investor
Medical Director
Diagnostic Test Interpretation (can be full-time or part-time, salaried, or independent consultant)
Hospital Administration
Financial Operations
Clinical Operations
Department Operations
Hospital Liaison to Medical School or Insurance Companies
Compliance Regulation, Technology Management
Wellness, Patient Education
Create Your Own Position
Long-Term Care
On-Site Director
Oversight
Patient Consultations
Accreditation
Insurance Industry
Business Executive
Clinical Operations
Medical Director
Review Specialist
Healthcare Provider Liaison
Healthcare Business—Healthcare Manufacturing Industry, Insurance, Venture Capital, Healthcare Management
Executive
Business Strategies
Management
Product Support

Benefits Management

Healthcare Financial Research

Healthcare Investment/Healthcare Financial Allocation

Marketing, Marketing Research

Sales

Technology

Direct Patient Care—Imaging, Surgical Equipment, Hospital Monitoring Equipment

Electronic Medical Records, Billing, and Ancillary Technology

Innovative Technology Implementation—Home Diabetes Monitoring, Artificial Limbs

Physician/Student Education

Medical School Teaching Director

Medical School Administration

University Teaching

Medical Entrance Examination and Certification Preparation

Continuing Medical Education

Medical Device Training

Technical Writing and Editing

Within a Medical Manufacturing or Medical Service Business

Independent Contractor

Working for a Medical Editing Provider

Public Health

Nonprofit Organization Director

Local Health Directives

Local Health Fund Allocation

Fund-Raising

Nontraditional Patient Care Alternatives

Moonlighting, Nocturnalist

Hospitalist

Telemedicine

Corporate Physician

Locum Tenens

Urgent Care

Visiting Physician

Disability Examinations

Concierge care

Drive-by Clinics

No More Patient Care

There are many ways to use your experience as a physician to pursue alternatives associated with medicine that do not directly involve patient care. These jobs require a degree of persistence, flexibility, and creativity on your part. You can use numerous qualifications that you have as a physician. Your hands-on experience with the practical aspects of patient care is priceless as you approach this avenue.

However, your clinical experience only plays a small direct role in attaining and flourishing in these broad-based positions. You will have to learn to work in a new type of environment and to develop new business skills or technical knowledge. You cannot completely ride on your medical school, residency, or even work experience to get you in the door or to keep you there. You may need to apply for positions in many companies, at many locations before you finally get a job offer. Recruiters are helpful in giving advice, but there are no companies looking for an MD who thinks he deserves a really great job just because he is a doctor and wants to try something new, or, worse, arrogantly believes that work that doesn't entail clinical practice must be easy.

As you will see in the following section, there are a variety of good choices out there for you if you want to use your foundation as an MD to embark on a different track. You already know that you have what it takes to get in to medical school and to be a good doctor. While the next step is by no means easy, you definitely have what it takes to find—and succeed at—satisfying nonclinical work. See Figure 5.2.

Scientific Research

Research physicians typically work either in universities or in industry. University positions vary and are often filled by doctors who continue to do some clinical work, although some university physicians devote their time completely to research. Some basic science researchers have a PhD in a science discipline, or a few years of supervised basic science research during or after residency training. University-employed research physicians generally take an initial research appointment with a salary agreement lasting for two to three years. After that time, physician researchers are expected to support their own salaries and research costs by securing grants. This requires writing grant proposals, as well as a track record of publications or other credibility-enhancing experience. A smaller minority of physicians works in clinical research. Grants for clinical research usually are given to doctors who have a well-respected clinical reputation and a large patient base.

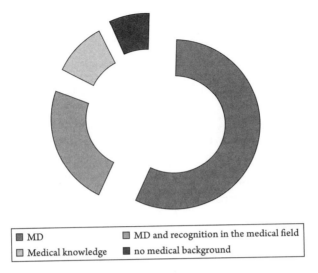

MD required: International Health, Risk Management, Regulatory Oversight, Insurance Work, Disability/Long Term Care, Laboratory Work, Industry Research, Patient Care

MD and distinguished background in the medical field required: Hospital Administration, Academic Research

Medical Knowledge needed: Public Health, Writing, Public Education, Teaching,

No medical background needed: Entrepreneurial, Policy, Technology, Business

Figure 5.1 What type of background do you need?

There are many prospects for doctors in commercial industry, such as pharmaceutical companies, biotechnology businesses, and medical device and equipment manufacturing. Most of these positions fall into either the categories of research and product development or business and administration. The research careers involve team-based basic science research or clinical research management. Basic science research in industry tends to be well funded and supported by a strong infrastructure. In contrast to university research, which is stereotypically characterized by a greater degree of academic freedom, industry investigative subject matter relates specifically to company product development objectives. Industry-based clinical research consists of coordinating patient-based studies to be conducted by practicing clinicians.

Government agencies such as the NIH and the Department of Defense are well-established organizations with prominent research sections. Positions at such agencies are highly prestigious, and often are filled by leaders in the field of medical research, or by promising research fellows.

Numerous small and large private medical research companies do medically related investigation for companies that outsource the task of scientific evaluation. For example, a nonmedical company that produces products with potential health implications, such as cosmetics or food, would hire a specialized research company to evaluate safety or applicability of products off-site. The results would then be used for product development and modification.

Medical Labs and Diagnostics

Medical labs and technology services are sometimes owned or supervised by physicians. Medical labs offer an opportunity for clinical interpretation, investment, or ownership. If your interest lies in marketing or efficient client service, you can use these abilities in imaging centers, neurodiagnostic testing facilities, blood laboratories, and genetic testing facilities, fertility services, or cord-blood storage facilities.

Most medical labs and imaging facilities are required to have a medical director. Some types of medical diagnostic testing sites must be staffed on-site by certified doctors to evaluate test results, supervise technician procedures, and provide accreditation for the facility. If you have an interest in pursuing opportunities in the medical lab world, it is absolutely critical to familiarize yourself with your state regulations regarding medical support facilities (such as accreditation requirements and self-referral policies), as these protocols have a major impact on your potential role as an investor, clinical director, or diagnostic test interpreter. I know several doctors who have obtained the qualification necessary for facility certification, which can make a physician almost indispensible to an operating facility.

Hospital Administration

There are usually positions for doctors in large clinics and hospitals in the area of hospital administration. This includes departmental leadership as well as hospital-wide responsibility in the capacities of financial operations and clinical organization. Additionally, large healthcare conglomerates, composed of several smaller institutions, typically maintain a level of clinical, financial, and operations management at each of the individual institutions in order to provide efficiency, uniformity, and support of healthcare services. Although prestigious positions often are filled by highly respected physicians already working within a particular healthcare institution and often take years to obtain, persistence and the flexibility to relocate may enable outsiders to find a place in this path.

Additional organizational administrative positions that are not traditionally as difficult to obtain include more behind-the-scenes work, such as institutional compliance regulation, case management, medical staff accreditation, medical technology management, and medical equipment supervision. When a nonphysician fulfills these roles they are compensated with a salary and benefits, and interestingly, when a physician performs the same duties, it is often expected to be on a volunteer basis. However, often a physician is well suited to do the job, and is better received by doctors and other medical personnel within the hospital. Therefore, it is useful for physicians to employ methods of applying for the paid positions, described in Chapter 7.

You also may be able to develop a new position in wellness promotion or outcomes assessment—two of the hottest areas of interest to healthcare organizations right now. If you can work with the administration to show how your proposed job can increase revenue, save money, or improve institutional ratings, you might create at least a part-time position for yourself. Similarly, community outreach is one of the latest areas that hospitals and healthcare institutions are using to expand their patient base and public reputation.

Long-Term Care

The day-to-day burden experienced by disabled patients in nursing homes and long-term-care facilities continues to require improvement. As a physician, you have options in this field, where you can make a significant difference in the lives of patients, their families, and their caregivers, by working in a long-term-care facility as a medical director or administrator. You could work in oversight at a state or county level for long-term-care facilities. This type of position could entail appraising compliance criteria that patient care institutions must follow. You could find alternative opportunities as an overseer for a government regulatory agency or a professional association.

If long-term-care work appeals to you, it is important to note that this is an area that is currently developing in a positive direction. There continues to be an expansion of rehabilitation facilities and day care facilities as well as substantial support systems for the handicapped. Additionally, the quality of care in such institutions is expected to improve due to determined patient advocacy efforts.

Insurance

The healthcare insurance industry offers many jobs that may require a persistent search, because they are not widely publicized. Such positions might also require travel or relocation. If you are interested in this type of business, you can work either directly for a health insurance company or for a consulting company that provides services to multiple insurance companies. There are full-time positions, such as a medical director or business executive, as well as part-time positions, such as medical advisor, MD peer reviewer, physician case manager, or appeals specialist. As an appeals specialist, you would evaluate appeals for procedures or medical conditions requiring physician review, while as a case manager, you would have a more long-term perspective over patient care. Your experience and degree are valuable to these companies not only for your practical work experience but also for credibility and, often, accreditation of the company itself. Entry level positions include those listed above, but other positions filled by experienced doctors include senior medical director, a role supervising medical directors and nursing staff, and chief medical officer, providing oversight over a wide sphere or division. A senior medical director, who hires most of the physicians within a leading healthcare review company explains that the credentialing process in peer review is similar to that of a hospital and that the utilization review and healthcare management system has stringent requirements and cannot serve as a retreat for bad doctors or doctors who have certification problems.

While there is often a stereotype of payers and regulators as the enemy of the medical establishment, there is a great deal of productive dialogue between physician organizations or physician specialty societies and the insurance industry or government agencies. Liaison roles for doctors dealing with regulation, payment, education, and numerous other issues often require travel and a great deal of background preparation, but often allow the flexibility to remain in clinical practice.

Part-time positions most often offer hourly wages, while full-time positions offer competitive salaries. Conflict-of-interest policies (such as working part-time in a consulting or insurance company while also seeing patients served by the insurance company, or consulting for more than one company) are typically clearly spelled out in physician contracts. If not, it is well worth it to bring up the subject, as these companies often merge or divide over the years, and your responsibilities may undergo modification as well. The insurance industry is mandated to respond to frequent changes in the economy and government regulation, often necessitating significant shifts in focus. This triggers the need for more jobs—such as outcomes assessment, compliance officer, and accreditation specialist—that you, as a physician, can fill.

Business

Most corporations or companies that produce or distribute healthcare products and services, such as imaging machines, hospital and surgical supplies, or patient rehabilitation equipment, have positions for physicians. As noted earlier, physicians are well suited for scientific research and product development. But within both the insurance industry and the healthcare manufacturing industry, your personal skills and interests may be more matched to marketing, management, business strategies, or even sales and product support. Lew Schwartz, MD, PhD, division vice president of absorbable stents at Abbot Laboratories, explains that there is a role for MDs in the area of medical liaison between product development and business. There are many doctors in numerous different functions in the health product industry.

If you are interested in health-care management strategies, many private organizations specialize in providing strategy and consulting to large health-care providers, health insurance companies, and employers. Companies often hire consultants for benefits management, the most costly of which is employee health benefits. Most businesses that employ large workforces are moving toward evaluating wellness initiatives, and their impact on overall company productivity and healthcare costs.

Additionally, you could consider using your background to look for options in business research organizations that evaluate the potential market for diverse healthcare products or devices, as well as the prospective financial return. Medical marketing companies conduct surveys for pharmaceutical companies or other health-related businesses. In the field of marketing, you could work for a marketing company that would handle presentation and promotion for a variety of health-related businesses or directly for a large medical business that has the need for its own marketing division.

You might choose to explore possibilities for nontraditional work with healthcare venture capital funds and organizations that consult with experts in the medical field to evaluate potential investments.

Brian Duncan, MD, a pediatric heart surgeon who had a busy clinical practice, was involved in research and publications on the niche topic of circulatory support for children. He became the principal investigator for a team working on mechanical circulatory support at Cleveland Clinic. As he led a team working on product development, he decided to get a business degree to understand the business aspects of product development and medical device commercialization. With his business and research background, he later became medical director of emerging businesses at Cleveland Clinic. In that role, he developed a relationship with a venture capital firm. While he describes the job of being a pediatric heart surgeon as a special opportunity to help patients and the "best job in the world," venture capital captured his imagination. He spent six months as an executive in residence at Arboretum Ventures, an Ann Arbor, Michigan–based venture capital firm that specializes in healthcare technology. This was an opportunity for Dr. Duncan to learn more about the business of venture capital and to see if the work environment was right for him. He subsequently transitioned to a permanent role and is currently a venture partner at Arboretum Ventures.

Dr. Duncan says that clinicians can contribute positively to the field of venture capital with multiple points of entry into these firms. An early career physician can enter as an associate, which provides increasing experience analogous to that obtained during clinical residency. This can allow a doctor entering the field to learn the business from the ground up. More senior level physicians might enter as venture partners, providing assistance with investment decision-making based on their experience in science and clinical medicine.

Business has traditionally been a field with vastly variable income levels, time demands, job descriptions, and ranges of responsibility. The field of business is so wide, that the term "business" is almost too general for most physicians to really get a grasp of. Dr. Duncan's story demonstrates that success in the field of business is attainable and that the depth of physician expertise and experience can bring an applicable skill into the business world. Several doctors who have transitioned into the investment and business world advised that education and expertise in business is not a rare commodity, but that experience and expertise in a science discipline combined with a business degree or business experience is a valuable background.

Technology

If you are skilled in technology, your background in medicine can uniquely position you as an expert in the implementation and interface between new technology and medicine. For example, new technologies that implement the tools necessary for surgery simulation training require both technological knowledge and an understanding of practical medicine. New equipment that provides better patient care must work in a way that is compatible with tools that have already been in use.

As the reliance on electronic medical records becomes both increasingly prevalent, yet disjointed, the need for more compatible systems of medical records management and practical application will inevitably grow. Expectations for remote access of patient records continue to increase, while the ethical and legal need for patient privacy remain essential. Medicare's new electronic medical record requirements for healthcare providers are due by 2014. Requirements such as these and their proposed incentives or penalties frequently change. As with other nonclinical medical areas, you would serve yourself well to know updated information regarding regulations if you plan to search for opportunities in the technology arena. The inevitable improvements in maintaining and accessing patient data will continue to offer exciting possibilities for doctors interested in and skilled in technology.

Mark Estafanous, MD, an ophthalmologist from northeastern Ohio says that his single-specialty group was underwhelmed by the available Electronic Medical

Records options. He has an interest and skill in technology and programming and found EMR discussion sites on the Internet, chiefly to try to shop for a better program to purchase. But he found on the discussions, that some EMR programmers did not seem to tailor the programs to the patient physical exam structures that doctors needed. He was concerned that doctors would have to adapt their patient care habits to the EMR programs, rather than the EMR programs adapting to medically rational patient care needs. So he decided to write his own EMR program from scratch for his opthalmology group's use. After one of his partners mentioned the solution to an out-of-town ophthalmologist who had the same complaint about available EMRs, Dr. Estafanous sold his first Electronic Medical Records program to another single-specialty group. He learned of national conferences that can help supplement skills for EMR programmers and provide networking opportunities, but he still modestly states that his objective is to make the program as compatible with clinical practice for other physicians as possible.

His story illustrates how physicians can look at healthcare services from the inside rather than from the outside. It is a huge challenge to master a skill such as creating a software program "on the side." In Dr. Estafanous's case, he built the program while continuing full-time clinical practice. He admits that, while he is pleased with the final product, the dual role is extremely demanding. However, because of his clinical experience and his own understanding of the practical inadequacies of the available programs, his program was far more practical for fellow physicians.

Teaching

Clinical staff who have shown great skill in and dedication to teaching most often fill medical school administrative positions such as admissions dean, clinical skills program director, or teaching program director. If you are interested in one of these posts, it is helpful to have a good working association with the medical school administrative staff. Additionally, preliminary responsibilities can grow into a better-defined position, especially if peers and academic deans have the opportunity to get to know you and admire your work. You may be able to create your own position or lobby to expand your part-time position into something more substantial if you are able to provide a better service for the school or fill in a needed gap.

The dean of admissions at a prominent medical school began her involvement with medical school admissions by doing interviews for prospective medical students early in her career. She had been doing this out of interest, not necessarily eyeing a career modification. This grew into sitting on the admissions committee, a role that entailed a significant commitment of her time, but did not require modification of her clinical responsibilities. When she accepted an appointment as assistant dean of admissions, she made the choice to maintain a hybrid career instead of taking a full-time administrative position, and has continued this way even after her promotion as admissions dean, because she enjoys the practice of dermatology, and has not wanted to give it up. She admits that it can be difficult to maintain both functions, but credits her supportive staff with her ability to continue in clinical medicine while serving in administration.

This doctor's story demonstrates that even relatively early in a physician's career, demonstrating dedication and commitment to nonclinical functions can result in leadership positions. The fusion of a clinical career and another alternative career can be tricky due to the demands of work and the financial weight of clinical practice. Therefore, it takes planning and clear communication with both sides of the agreement in order to achieve a balance.

If your interest is in residency and training education, your national specialty board has a growing need for uniform, updated, and relevant educational program learning objectives. As healthcare specialties continue to expand and intensify their recertification requirements, there is an increasing need for national specialty board certification measures.

On a similar note, you may be able to teach college-level health science classes. This can also allow you to take classes at a reduced tuition in a field that interests you. These jobs most often pay less than clinical positions, but offer vacations, reasonable work hours, and exposure to an enriching academic environment. In addition, you might consider teaching preparation courses for medical entrance examinations, boards, and other certification examinations, either on your own, or as a part of an established test preparation site.

Physician Education

Internet companies that provide CME for medical professionals or healthcare information sites are relatively new and are evolving, as many Internet-only companies are. Therefore, if you have an interest in patient education or in education for healthcare professionals, it would be to your advantage to become acquainted with the websites and make every effort to contact the editors by e-mail as well as by phone to inquire about positions. Often university staff edit these sites voluntarily, but as they continue to become more popular, more paying positions may open up.

As new medical devices and treatment methods become available, practicing clinicians take courses to learn how to perform new procedures in order to offer their patients better treatment options. You could consider becoming certified to teach physicians and other healthcare professionals how to use a new device and to continue to provide support for those physicians as they become acquainted with new techniques and devices.

Writing

As a physician, you can edit medical informational articles for accuracy for a variety of audiences. If you are very organized and willing to take on a big project, you might consider medical textbook writing or editing. If you have writing talent, you could find work writing grants or proposals either for an established company or as an independent contractor. Many pharmaceutical companies and government agencies rely on medical writing specialists for professional correspondence.

There are positions for medical writers within companies that manufacture medical devices or other healthcare products and services. Depending on the company, the need for writing technical medical plans, customer information, or patient materials, may be provided by either a branch within the company or outsourced to a specialized medical writing specialist. Due to the relatively low overhead, medical writing is an opportunity that physicians can also do as independent contractors.

Public Education

Patient education and public education are areas that many physicians, such as Roxanne Sukol, MD, who runs a popular healthcare blog, *Your Health Is on Your Plate*, feel compelled to do for the good of their patients and the general public. Dr. Sukol says that her blog was a natural transition after she had regularly written a news column for an organic food CSA (community-supported agriculture) co-op. She says that in her office she noticed interesting things about her patients. For example, she observed that there was an increased association of diabetes in spouses of patients with diabetes. She thought that this must be related to nutritional factors. She began to learn about, and then teach about, nutrition management. She says that as she wrote about these subjects, visits to her blog exploded. She viewed it as a vehicle to teach patients, and her speaking engagements and consulting requests were not an intentional consequence of her efforts but an opportunity to continue to educate the public.

Dr. Sukol has changed her clinical practice to match her overall public education goals and she currently works in the Wellness Institute at the Cleveland Clinic developing programs that can improve health in a global way. One of her objectives is to change the paradigm of diabetes diagnosis with the objective of earlier stage diabetes prevention.

Fresh venues for writing patient communication brochures and educational information for the public can be found through public health associations, patient support organizations, and for-profit companies that provide healthcare products.

However, it is important to note that due to the abundance of healthcare sites, articles, and blogs on the Internet, there are numerous websites that do not pay writers. Indeed, without a recognized background in publications, it may be extremely difficult to expect pay in return for writing a good healthcare article. A start would be contributing articles for a health sites and reading all feedback, as well as following how many hits your article receives. This feedback can help you to improve your writing and gauge readers' expectations and interests.

Oversight

There are many state and national regulatory agencies for compliance oversight, outcomes management, and regulatory certification administration. The medical field, as we all know, is abundant with mandates, and few are truly qualified to assess compliance, while even fewer are able to assist in making compliance manageable.

Typically, a committee of appointed positions within a state medical society or national specialty association produces recommendations for health conditions, such as immunization recommendations or prenatal screening tests. State or county regulatory agencies use these physician-approved recommendations as one of several tools for policy in conjunction with consideration of resource availability.

You may consider applying for a position within an oversight committee, such as the Joint Commission for Accreditation for Hospital Organizations, or the Residency Review Committee. But, as these positions are few, a preliminary step could be aiming for an appointed position in your state or specialty association. This will give you access to the people you will need to meet and also will ultimately improve your qualifications for a paid position.

Risk Management and Legal Work

In the area of risk management, you can play a role in improving healthcare quality by working within a healthcare system or with a risk management business. Most hospitals require professional clinical staff to participate in risk management educational programs. Additionally, risk management staff can offer much needed clinician support and advice.

It is worth mentioning that litigation review and testimony are the most commonly documented nonclinical fields for physicians. Few physicians do such work full-time, as clinical practice is often a prerequisite and the availability of litigation assignments may be variable over time. One physician expressed that she felt somewhat unhappy with herself after one such job because she found herself speaking to a jury of upstanding, educated citizens who did not have a medical background. She says that she had concerns that the well-meaning individuals could be potentially manipulated due to the highly technical nature of the case.

A litigation attorney in a fairly small city tells me that he has difficulty when it comes to finding physicians in his town to testify against one another. He says that due to a combination of the reasonable cost of living and the local professional camaraderie among doctors in his town, he must search for expert witnesses out of state. He says that due to the higher costs associated with contracting out-of-town doctors, he tries to avoid using expert witnesses unless absolutely necessary. Additionally, he shares that most physicians whom he hires to do expert witness work take substantial cautions to keep the fact that they have done this type of work hush-hush among patients and other doctors. He says that he is careful to avoid hiring physicians who have been heavily involved in litigation work, as this can lead to marked criticism of the physician as an opportunist, from the opposing side, actually weakening his case.

Certainly, not every opportunity for legal work is harmful, and some can contribute to patients' rights. But, as a general rule, work that may alienate others, or work that you do not show pride in doing, can set the stage for regret later on. I spoke to an attorney who believes that MDs have unrealistic expectations regarding compensation. This attorney clarifies that the true goal of legal work lies in helping those who have been wronged, and that people who have suffered from injuries need a compassionate advocate. She explains that sometimes doctors believe in a myth that money is being "thrown around" in the legal world. She states that medical expert work is neither exciting nor easy and that doctors provide her with very detailed well-documented data that requires a great deal of painstaking preparation and time, with moderate compensation.

One physician, an internist living in a region with a high cost of living, says that he works as an independent contractor for auto insurance companies, who ask him to evaluate accident injury claims for medical validity. He explains that this is a way for him to gain a supplemental salary without adding clinical hours, while avoiding the problem of potentially alienating other physicians.

Public Health

Such positions as free clinic director or city or county public health director are few and far between. Realistically, this type of job search includes meeting people in positions to appoint such jobs, and making them aware of your experience and goals while also asking about their goals for their organization. These meetings may introduce you to opportunities with similar organizations.

Nonprofit organizations and foundations or societies for various medical conditions, such as the Multiple Sclerosis Society or cancer foundations, can be a source of employment for physicians in the arena of fund-raising or in allocation of services and funds. Positions might begin as goal-oriented projects addressing specific public health concerns such as teen pregnancy, domestic abuse, or community drug education. If you have such interest, it is worthwhile to become adept at writing grants to support this work and to learn to effectively measure outcomes of such programs.

Additionally, cities, counties, and communities often have community health goals and physician oversight for health and safety programs and objectives. Some school systems may have a physician serving in the role of constructing schoolwide and student health recommendations. Public health organizations differ among cities and counties and do not necessarily follow the same pattern from one location to another. Some cities may have health directors, while others might not and may rely on volunteers to construct local public health policies and recommendations.

Policy

Some physicians go on to pursue politics or healthcare policy. The option of running for elected office requires a tremendous amount of time, planning, dedication, and persistence. One needs to have thick skin and to be able to get up and try, try, try again. These pursuits are not for the easily crushed, and also must be prepped for while you have another paying job, as it may take years to establish an income—which may disappear after the next election. A number of physicians transition into this role quite effectively, as experience in working with patients so closely provides a true opportunity for physician politicians to really understand their constituents, and their day-to-day concerns.

If you are interested in politics and public policy but not in the prospect of becoming the possible recipient of the inevitable political bad-mouthing that accompanies a political campaign, there are several other options that are more low-key. Political campaign managers, government staff, health policy advisors, and political speechwriters can play a fundamental role in policy without the publicity of elected positions. Additionally, healthcare advocacy is most often unpaid and sporadic but can provide a background for a full-time job.

Clinician Resources and Support

There is a role for doctors in companies that provide billing and medical record services. As a practicing physician, your more valuable role will be in contributing to tools that make doctors' jobs easier. Some established businesses provide physician resources, and the best way for these businesses to supply meaningful services is for a doctor who has struggled with day-to-day patient care to play a pivotal role in the process. This arena can be as varied as you can imagine, from providing medical billing services to medical staffing to marketing to physician recruitment.

Shelly Brown, an orthopedic surgeon, was unsatisfied with surgical positioning devices for some of her surgical procedures. She already had a working relationship with the surgical device equipment product representative at her hospital, who often was present during surgical procedures to assess demand for products and to help physicians use some surgical devices. With his help, she contacted the company and arranged to have them make a surgical positioning device that she designed. The product is sold to other orthopedic surgeons and hospitals, is made to order, and Dr. Brown has a contract to share in the profit from the device that she designed that the product company manufactures and markets.

Often physicians have to take initiative to make clinical practice more effective. In this example, Dr. Brown's incentive was primarily to have the product, a device with relatively little turnover, for her own use. However, physicians may design a product with higher turnover and wider use if they see a deficiency in available products.

Out of the Box

Given the rapid advancement of technology and the globally connected economy, the area of telemedicine is likely to expand and change dramatically. Telemedicine began primarily as a way to provide radiology services to remote areas that do not have enough patient volume to support or attract on-site radiologists. As the technological infrastructure grew, the field of telemedicine expanded to include imaging procedures such as cardiac echo, ICU monitoring, and now clinical visits. Lorraine Millas, a recruiter for a telemedicine company that provides neurological services, explains that the demand for telemedicine clinical consultation services is growing. In some situations, a doctor may cover a wide geographical area, and require telemedicine to properly evaluate patients for situations such as TPA evaluation, when time is of critical importance. She explains that there are many rural areas in the United States with a deficit of physicians. Additionally, she conveys that telemedicine staffing companies are an efficient way for doctors to find telemedicine work. This is due to the fact that the volume at many of the hospitals that contract for telemedicine may be low, allowing physician work shifts that combine physician coverage for a few hospitals that may not even be geographically near each other.

Expectations for healthcare quality continue to increase, even for those with remote access. In order to meet higher expectations in the future, triage, and even treatment by properly certified doctors, will need to be provided in nontraditional ways. Of course, as medicine moves more toward evidence-based payment structures, we can anticipate the continued evaluation of the *value* of new options such as telemedicine. Doctors can certainly take the opportunity to play a major role in the assessment of the usefulness of new services.

International medical care typically offers little to no income, but can be an enjoyable way to see the world, and use your advanced skills to serve others, to appreciate medicine from a completely different viewpoint, and learn more about your specialty. There is a need for all medical specialties, not just primary care or infectious disease specialists, which is a stereotype that discourages some physicians from approaching this alternative. Organizations such as the World Health Organization, Doctors without Borders, and many religious and community groups can help you in arranging your trip. International medical work can be a full-time career, a short-term volunteer stint, or a physician-led project geared toward a specific population or goal. Short-term assignments generally are best with a well-established group. Physicians who have had years of experience could be assigned to disaster relief roles, where a working understanding of the pressing needs of international health is crucial. For those who demonstrate years of true dedication, an administrative role in international health can provide a stable job and the ability to have an impact on global health for the underserved.

Purchit Lacuesta, MD, a practicing internist in Chicago, has been to Mexico, Cambodia, Kenya, and Guatemala to do medical mission work and describes each trip as unique. She says of Guatemala, "it was cool because we seriously had clinic in the rain forest. The hardest thing about these trips is the language barrier. I can't help but concentrate on what people are saying even if it is not English, and then listen to the translation. I try to do both, just to see if I can tell if the info exchanged is accurate. It is not foolproof, but I still try. It is still mentally tiring. The medical part is actually easier, because there is only a finite amount that you can do." She also describes working at an orphanage in Kenya, "I slowly made it through the orphanage and made recommendations on treatment so that when contributions came in, they could prioritize who got what kind of care. The more doctors use their talents out in the field, the better. I think that it is hard for people to just get out there to do something," she explains, echoing the concept that initiating something is often one of the greatest challenges.

Other unique, out-of-the-box possibilities for doctors include directing a health or science museum, producing or directing public health education videos, or writing medical fiction.

Patient Care Without the Hassles

Some physician opportunities involve patient care, but fall outside the definition of a traditional full-time clinical practice. In these situations you can limit some of the hassles of daily patient care responsibilities, on-call coverage, billing, documentation, off-duty expectations, and so forth. The most common of these practice options is locum tenens work. This is clinical work with a short-term contract and very clear expectations. It is an option that many physicians have elected for various reasons. Some physicians do locum tenens work during the phase of establishing a new practice in order to earn an income while still building a patient base. I know several physicians who took on locum tenens work after leaving a job to give themselves time to look for a suitable position without the financial pressure of a rushed timetable.

Most locum tenens companies have an agreement with physicians to provide work opportunities with clear expectations, competitive pay, and malpractice insurance, plus assistance with out-of-state licensing applications and fees. The majority of locums work requires travel to underserved rural areas, although occasionally temporary positions become available in large cities. The locums placement companies have their own recruiters who will listen to your current situation and explain the options they have for you and what those jobs pay.

You should always be honest regarding your concerns about board qualifications as well as state licensing and any past disciplinary action. Locums recruiters have experience with the medical licensing process and they are obligated to provide quality doctors to the healthcare establishments they work with. Recruiters can give you sound information regarding any regulatory issues and what you can do about these protocols, even if you are not qualified to do work through the specific recruiter that you have been in contact with.

A similar option, moonlighting, also offers temporary work with short-term contracts and responsibilities. This option typically offers primarily nighttime and weekend hours and it can allow you to maintain an income while you shift into your next career phase. As with locum tenens, just as you are not obligated by a long-term contract, neither is your employer. You may be needed only briefly until a full-time position is filled. However, in some hospitals and health systems moonlighting physicians are a permanent physician-staffing feature. A newer type of hybrid between moonlighting and hospitalist work has been described as nocturnalist, a physician who takes a permanent position to work hospital night shifts only.

Similar opportunities that can enable you to work as a clinical physician with fewer strings attached include: staffing an urgent care center; performing patient consultations in rehabilitation or long-term-care facilities; patient care at an Indian reservation; working as a visiting doctor; hospice care; long-term-care facility consultant; performing disability, medical-legal, or insurance examinations; and even becoming a prison physician. There is a new trend of concierge medicine, which can enable a physician to take fewer patients, with varied payment plans. As the public becomes increasingly alarmed about healthcare access, there is an increase in demand for such services, although the benefit to patients has not yet been well documented. While I have commented on the overproliferation of rules and regulations in medical care, it is important to watch out for opportunities in which rules may be lacking or situations such as concierge care, in which paying patients might feel that they have the right to demand unusual or unsafe medical services.

There is also a growing trend among large corporations to employ physicians on-site to care for employee health needs. These companies typically need either full-time doctors or part-time physician independent contractors, effectively reducing sick leave for company employees and providing continuity of care. It is worth noting that you can proactively propose a new clinic setup in a large company that does not yet have one in place, if you can provide numbers supporting the cost savings and efficiency of your proposed setup.

Advantages of positions such as locums or other temporary clinical work include good hourly pay, flexible work hours, and covered malpractice—without concern of a tail payment if you stop working at a specific location or establish a completely nonclinical career altogether. You also will not be faced with the difficulty of having to officially resign from a practice that has been counting on you. Coverage of the cost of malpractice and malpractice tail cost by your employer is customary, but it is still extremely important for you to ask about all malpractice insurance policy issues and tail responsibility, and to review all contracts in detail before you begin work.

This type of work can really be a good way to transition into an alternative field, while maintaining an income doing what you are already qualified to do. Some doctors enjoy the flexibility and freedom of these types of practice arrangements long-term. See Figure 5.3.

Conclusion

You may decide to leave medicine altogether. If you take that route, remember that you will enter into a field where your specific degree is not explicitly valuable.

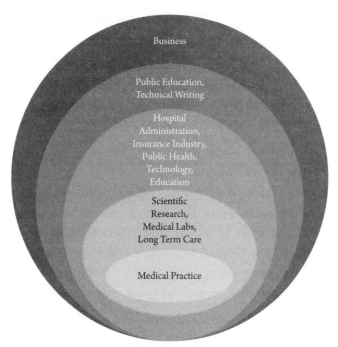

Figure 5.2 How similar are alternative fields to medical practice?

Still, the fact that you have an advanced degree, and that you have gained personal skills and profession skills, while you trained and worked as a physician, is significant. That is what you need to emphasize, both to potential employers, and to yourself. You might decide to start your own business in a field that has nothing to do with medicine, such as a design company. You might decide to become a fiction writer or a real estate developer. Whatever you choose, you may need to obtain more education or instruction—either to gain certification and make yourself more marketable or simply to learn the new material in a setting where you will get useful feedback.

If your area of interest does not demand, value, or even use your experience as a physician, is that a reason to avoid pursuing that field? What if you already know that you do not want to have anything to do with medicine and you will not use your background as leverage? This is a tough question that only you can answer.

You might, and likely will, start at a more junior level if you choose a field in which medicine does not have any relevance. As noted in Chapter 4, how you choose to spend your working hours has to do with time, money, status, serving others, or any of a number of other considerations. You have to decide which factors are most important to you. And in making those choices, you will certainly have to give up some potential benefits.

There are numerous opportunities for you if you would like to leave clinical medicine to do something else. Once you decide which direction you want
to take based on your personal and professional interests and your obligations,
you can begin to take the right steps to ensure that you find the right job for
yourself.

Numbers: The Taboo Nobody Wants to Talk About. Shhh … It's All in Here

While many physicians want to leave clinical practice, the mystery surrounding the financial viability of alternative options often inhibits doctors from initiating the move into another position. And, for many reasons, it can be difficult to determine the practical and economic implications of a professional change for physicians.

There are a few contributing factors to the enigmatic nature of finding reliable salary information. The basic fact that it is improper to ask someone how much money he or she earns makes it challenging to obtain figures. People may be prone to misleading others about income, either out of a need to appear more successful than they really are, a measured cautiousness to deter jealousy, or simply because everyone is entitled to privacy. There is wide variation in published data about salaries and it can be difficult to ascertain where the information comes from. Nevertheless, accurate figures are critical for most people who are considering committing time and energy to a job search and possibly giving up a secure position. Therefore, I have researched reliable information about projected income in alternative fields for doctors. This material was obtained using a combination of interviews with physicians who have worked in the jobs described at varied levels of experience, physician directors who hire and search for doctors to fill a range of posts, and knowledgeable recruiters who have placed hundreds of jobs, and my own extensive evaluation of numerous job listings with wide regional representation (including phone calls to the companies listing the jobs), as well as authoritative published data.

Each individual doctor may view the financial consequences of leaving clinical medicine completely differently. Doctors hold variable levels of interest in economic matters to begin with. There is no doubt that some MDs enjoy playing an active role in their investments and money management, while others prefer to maintain a more hands-off approach. For doctors who have already had long careers and have built a safety net of savings that they can use to invest and support themselves, salary from nonmedical work may be less of a concern. However, the majority of doctors need to continue to earn a living while transitioning into an alternate career and must continue to support themselves and their families with their nontraditional jobs for years to come.

Guidelines for calculation of exit costs certainly are important as well. The estimated time and energy required in making this transition is a significant factor. Making a career change, unlike the establishment of a first career, is usually done at a stage in life when there are already other time-consuming demands, such as family and unconcluded job responsibility.

How Many Doctors Are There?

According to the US Bureau of Labor Statistics (USBLS; data cited in this chapter available at http://www.bls.gov/bls/website-policies.htm), physicians held about 661,400 jobs in 2008. This number reflects the number of physicians who were directly employed as doctors. Predictions of physician shortage and physician surplus have been dramatically variable and contradictory. The projected demand for physicians is a particularly difficult number to understand because there are so many variables such as better medical treatments, growing population, poor health of the uninsured, the role of physician extenders, and numerous other unpredictable factors. If we deem the anticipated projected employment of physicians in 2018 to be 805,500 per the US Bureau of Labor Statistics, while there are approximately 19,000 medical school graduates per year (currently, there are 159 medical schools in the United States, each with an average of approximately 120 graduates awarded an MD or DO degree per year) with an average career span of 40 years, then the supply of doctors would be about 760,000, which is lower than the demand.

Why does the number of physicians and projected employment estimates matter if you are considering leaving clinical practice? It matters if you are looking for a job that only a doctor can fill or for a job that is best filled by a physician. Given that there is an increase in physicians demanding reasonable work hours, a slowing down of direct patient care done during work hours due to increasing documentation, the number of physicians required to do the same amount of patient care work will likely increase. If the trend of increasing mandates and raising qualification criteria as a solution for quality enhancement continues, the demand for your credentials as a physician may swell even in the nonclinical setting. The pool of available physicians qualified to fill posts requiring difficult-to-attain medical licensure qualifications remains limited due to the number of years it takes to qualify for medical licensure and certification. This can be an advantage for you as you make a transition using your expertise and credentials.

How Many Doctors Are in Nontraditional Medical Careers? Is There Too Much Competition?

Numerous websites and articles in financial magazines are devoted to the topic of career changes for professionals. Actual numbers are impossible to track down for any profession, and even more so for doctors. April Confessore, a recruiter with Infinite Talent Medical Staffing, says that while she recruits exclusively for clinical work, she receives frequent calls from MDs inquiring about nonclinical opportunities. The specialized physician placement headhunters with whom I spoke acknowledged a growing number of inquiries from physicians looking for nonclinical employment, but were unable to estimate numbers or whether supply and demand for physicians in nontraditional roles are in synch. There are not currently recruiting companies with a focus on placing physicians in nonclinical fields. This is largely due to two factors. First, there is a high demand for clinical physician placement, which keeps recruiters busy. Second, the types of companies that might need a physician to work in a non clinical job are vastly diverse, as described in Chapter 5.

It is difficult to reliably determine how many physicians actually want to leave clinical medicine but cannot do so, versus how many physicians want to leave clinical medicine yet have made no attempts to do so. Given the experiences of the physicians who shared their insight for this book, it appears that while it is not easy, conditions are favorable for a physician who is dedicated to finding nontraditional work to find a suitable position. I have spoken to numerous physicians who expressed an interest in changing careers but have made no attempts to begin the process, due to the hurdles examined in Chapter 3. Getting started is the principal limiting factor, primarily because as noted earlier, there is no recognized system of placement but rather more of a "make your own rules" path. There is no "nonclinical" box on the match form that you can fill in. The guidelines in Chapter 7 provide direction on how to obtain a nonclinical position and, in reality, demonstrate a more exhaustive effort than most physicians have actually had to put into the transition. A reasonable degree of persistence materializes into concrete opportunities.

Richard Smith, MD, MBA, a senior medical director with a large review company, says that there is a consistent need for doctors in the insurance industry. There are numerous opportunities for physicians both within insurance companies, and in companies that provide outsourcing services to healthcare plans. Ashraf Hanna, MD, PhD, a vice president of commercial finance at Genentech; and Lew Schwartz, MD, a division vice president at Abbot laboratories; explain that there is a consistent and constant need for physicians in the pharmaceutical and biotechnology industry, in many different capacities. Many of the other physicians I spoke with have been able to find entry-level positions in the well-established pharmaceutical industries and healthcare insurance or management fields shortly after completing residency.

The typical doctor maintained a full-time clinical job during the nonclinical job search. Most physicians initiated meaningful contact with between five and fifteen companies, including thorough, specific job inquiries targeted toward a person in an influential level of the company, and maintained dedicated follow-up. Personal interviews were arranged in approximately one-third of the contacts and subsequently resulted in job offers at least half of the time. The physicians who made the effort to look for nonclinical jobs typically explained to me that they received several job offers, as well as some rejections, within six months of the first job search.

The overall feedback I have gotten from industry recruiters is that recruiters need to pursue doctors for industry openings and that some physician openings can take months for companies to fill, even in this current economic atmosphere. Entry-level jobs, which, of course, pay less on the average than more senior level positions, are available. There appear to be more positions for nontraditional work opportunities than there are physicians actively looking to fill such jobs. However, because there are many companies in different industries, and because there is a great patchiness in need based on timing, it will most likely take committed effort on the part of a physician to *identify* an existing opening and to get on the radar of recruiters. Posts for higher-level jobs require experience either in medical practice or in entry-level nonclinical positions and, while there are prospects for applicants, these opportunities more often require relocation, frequent travel, and are usually filled by a process involving a candidate search, rather than the other way around.

If you are determined, you should not be under the impression that you are in competition with other MDs for scarce opportunities. Your qualifications, and how well you present yourself, will be the primary factor in opening doors for you. In fact, everyone I spoke with who hires physicians for nonclinical jobs told me that they often opt to leave positions open if there is not a qualified candidate, rather than filling positions with mediocre candidates.

Clinical Practice

The United States Bureau of Labor Statistics data reports that in 2008, physicians had total median annual compensation of $186,044. There is marked variation in physician income based on regional differences, size of the city, practice model, and medical specialty. In general, physician reimbursement is higher in rural towns than in large cities, higher in the Southwest, and lower in coastal regions. Typically, positions in large institutions or in academic settings offer lower salaries than in private practices. Procedural-based specialties, which often require more years of training, generally pay more than nonprocedural specialties. Benchmarks of traditional practice monetary compensation are useful for evaluating the numerical factors involved in the transition to another career.

Due to proposed Medicare payment cuts of approximately 20% for physician services, the above numbers may change over the next several years. Estimations of the impact of such cuts are complicated, difficult, and often unreliable. Given that a physician may be forced to accept 20% less payment for patient care services while support staff salary and benefits, malpractice insurance costs, space and equipment rental, and other costs traditionally increase with inflation, a 20% reimbursement rate decrease (gross decrease) can be expected to decrease net income by more than 20%.

There are some notable trends in the differences between physician compensation for clinical work and nonclinical compensation. Nonclinical salary ranges are wider than physician salaries. Unlike in clinical practice, reputable specialty training and high-level clinical skill may contribute slightly to making a doctor more coveted by nonclinical companies but does not translate into a higher salary for that physician. Similarly, distinctive physician specialists that perform uncommon procedures, such as transplant surgery, may not be more numerically valued in the nonclinical setting than more prevalent specialties. Regional differences in physician salary are markedly less significant in the nonclinical setting than in the clinical setting, as it is often difficult for hospitals to recruit clinical physicians to work in some regions of the country. But the availability of nonclinical jobs is typically limited to large metropolitan cities or locations where medical product companies are located, in contrast to clinical care, where the need for MDs is roughly proportional to patient population.

How Much Do Alternative Jobs Pay? See Figure 6.1.

Using Your Medical License

Locums, moonlighting, and telemedicine generally pay hourly, sometimes with minimum monthly work requirements in order to justify the cost of malpractice insurance coverage and out-of-state licensing fees. The doctors and recruiters that I spoke with about this type of work highlighted that placement companies look for physicians with a reputable record regarding licensing and malpractice. Given that an MD has met the formal requirements of the job, most physicians who want to do this type of work are able to find positions. Recruiters for moonlighting and locums positions, however, stressed that it may be necessary to apply for several positions due to fluid company demand for physicians. But,

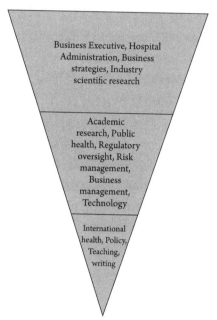

Figure 6.1 How much do alternative jobs pay?

given the straightforward nature of the application process, this has not been viewed by MDs as a cumbersome process. Lorraine Millas of NeuroCall, Inc., says that there is a constant need to fill telemedicine positions, as so many hospitals, particularly in rural areas, are turning to this method of physician staffing.

The pay varies, principally depending on the medical specialty. For example, radiologists typically earn between $150 and $250 per hour, while primary care physicians and medical specialists, such as neurologists, normally earn approximately $55–$110 per hour. Anesthesiologists, surgeons, and other specialists generally can expect compensation between $100 and $200 per hour for telemedicine, moonlighting, or similar work. Another factor that plays into the hourly salary is the location of the work. Clinical patient care in rural and underserved locations generally pays more than in larger cities, which have a larger pool of available physicians. It is worth noting that residents in training are also occasionally offered moonlighting opportunities, and that the compensation falls at the lowest end of this spectrum, and sometimes lower, depending on the requirements of the residency program.

Similar options that reimburse at comparable hourly rates include emergency medicine or urgent care staffing, which usually are more accessible to emergency medicine and primary care trained physicians, rather than specialists. Hospice care and home healthcare work is generally less commonly needed, demand for physicians tends to exceed the supply. Several doctors have mentioned to me that they do disability examinations, which is also in demand. This type of work requires time-consuming paperwork, a frequent physician complaint, but the paperwork can be more efficient for doctors who do a high volume, and employ staff who are acquainted with the system.

Clinical review, peer review, or case management, either in a hospital or insurance company setting is another hourly job that requires licensed physicians. The compensation falls anywhere from $100 to $200 per hour, depending on the type of work and the company and does not typically differ based on physician medical specialty. Peer review involves pharmacology or radiology management, hospitalization or procedural preauthorization, and case management. Physicians generally work in their area of clinical expertise, and there are jobs available, with many interested physician applicants.

Legal work can pay hourly, with rare instances of full-time physician employment in large law firms. Hourly rates for case review and expert witness testimony depend on the experience of the physician, the reputation of the institution that employs the physician, and most markedly, the region of the country. Rates per hour can vary from $75 to $225, and the higher range is often reserved for those coming from a health system with a strong institutional reputation. Often, the physician's employer maintains the rights to collect the litigation review fees, and may allot a prenegotiated percentage to physicians. If you have a strong interest in the legal field, you may want to consider beginning with SEAK, an organization that provides expert witness training for physicians.

Science and Industry

Basic science research careers, either in the academic or industry setting, require a background in research either as a PhD or as a basic science fellow. Academic positions require meaningful publications and a strong aptitude for writing grants. These jobs are only open to highly qualified research physicians, who may have to apply for positions at several different academic institutions or businesses. Even after securing a job, academic research physicians must continue to actively pursue funding and grants to support research and salary, whereas industry physicians do not.

Doctors in university research positions concur that entry-level jobs for basic science research physicians typically pay $100,000 per year to $180,000 per year. Variation in salary based on medical specialty tends to be more prevalent in academics than in industry, because clinical departments often contribute to the research budget in a university. Starting salaries and raises follow specific parameters within each individual institution and department in the academic setting. The potential salary for an academic research position is customarily slightly lower than that of a clinical practicing physician in the same specialty within the same institution.

The expected salary in industry-based research depends on experience. In industry, while some specialists may be in demand for recruitment at certain times, depending on a new product, a doctor's medical specialty is less of a distinguishable income factor among physicians within a company than it is in the combination clinical setting of a research university. Recruiters and physicians who hire doctors in industry positions consistently echo that starting salaries for entry-level physician jobs, such as clinical monitoring or marketing, without a great deal of clinical or research experience are in the range of $100,000 per year to $120,000 per year. Physicians who have experience in clinical medicine or basic science research generally earn higher starting salaries, in the range of $150,000 per year to $250,000 per year, and, as would be expected, hold higher levels of responsibility than less experienced doctors.

Dr. Mahmoud has evaluated many physician candidates for pharmaceutical positions during his tenure at Merck. He says that physicians play a critical role in the pharmaceutical industry. In fact, he says, the chairman of Merck in the late 1980s and early 1990s was a physician. Dr. Mahmoud says that industry has a clear understanding of staffing needs and looks for physicians that can specifically fill those responsibilities. He shares that the positions he was involved in recruiting for were fairly high level, including enlisting physician staff to help him launch new vaccines. He says that he received many applications from MDs and that, at Merck, his section did not hire whatever came their way but rather searched actively for qualified candidates with a proven track record of scientific experience or health policy.

But, he states that while his own industry needs required him to seek out highly qualified and experienced MDs, there are positions for physicians in industry at different levels. For example, entry-level positions include clinical monitors for clinical trials. He adds that doctors are needed in varied formats in the pharmaceutical industry, from marketing to research and development, to policy, to top-level positions. Dr. Mahmoud is encouraging regarding the chances of a qualified physician finding a role in industry. Many physicians reiterated the point that there is a constant but fluctuating need for doctors in the healthcare product industry. There is room for all specialties and different roles that doctors can fill.

Anticipated rungs of salary increases are higher for researchers in the business setting over time than in the university setting. However, there are generally more benefits in the academic setting, such as retirement plans and health and disability benefits. Dr. Schwartz explains that the method of payment is different in industry than in clinical practice or academic medicine, with incentives, a bonus structure, and stock options often equal to, or more than, the established salary. A significant difference noted by several physicians in industry, is that there may be a severance package, which typically does not exist for physicians in the clinical world.

Job security traditionally has been more stable for doctors in the academic setting than in the business setting. Dr. Schwartz also emphasizes that there is no job security in industry, in sharp contrast to clinical medicine, where there is high demand for practicing physicians of all specialties. He says that companywide changes in strategy can result in buyouts or layoffs. Ashraf Hanna, MD, PhD, vice president of commercial finance at Genentech explains, however, that when small companies dissolve, resulting in job loss, a physician can find a similar position at another company, because industry employed physicians are well aware of mergers and buyouts in their field, which often allows for transfer into a new job when such changes occur. Often, doctors in these situations must be flexible regarding geographic location.

Physicians who have achieved a high level of recognition either in the clinical, research, or administrative realm usually fill executive positions. Filling these jobs often entails a corporate search process, and the pay is, of course, higher. There is more than one possible route for a physician to move up to an executive or medical director position in the pharmaceutical, biotechnology, or insurance industry. MDs who excel in their entry-level nonclinical roles can progress to higher-level positions while remaining at the same company or moving to another one.

Administration

Government posts for administrative physicians typically pay salaries equivalent to a nonprocedural specialty in academics, in the range of $90,000 to $150,000 per year. Government positions usually require some travel, but not as much travel as jobs in the for-profit industries, such as health insurance organizations or medical product manufacturers.

Hospital administrative positions, such as chief medical officer, offer dramatically variable compensation, often depending on the size and financial health of the specific healthcare organization. Typically, a high-level administrative position in a small- to medium-sized hospital compensates at least slightly more than compensation for a practicing physician of that specialty within the hospital or healthcare system. However, MDs with broad level financial responsibility for a large healthcare institution can earn several times the amount of the highest paid clinical physician in a given department or institution.

Positions with niche areas of responsibility, or jobs that do not require an MD, such as quality assurance and risk management, also vary per institution. Often such positions are not full-time roles and are filled by doctors who continue to do clinical work. Generally, a physician with these added responsibilities maintains the same level of earnings as when in full-time clinical practice. Several physicians explained to me that they negotiated a decrease in clinical requirements with the hospital system that benefited from their additional work related to administration. Few doctors have been successful in negotiating additional pay for extra duties, typically using the strategy that additional pay to a physician already in the system is more efficient than hiring a new full-time manager and paying that manager for benefits as well as salary. For full-time administrative jobs that are not executive level, such as corporate compliance or risk management, a physician who has not previously held a clinical position in the hospital generally should expect to be compensated similarly to a non-MD manager, in the range of $80,000 per year to $100,000 per year.

Teaching

Physicians who teach at the medical school level are largely uncompensated financially, unless they hold a significant administrative role. A typical medical school has about ten to fifteen physician administrative deans. In most administrative medical school posts there is a well-established salary structure. High-level dean appointments generally offer more room for negotiating a package, including an infrastructure to support a vision for growth.

Other teaching roles besides medical school teaching can also offer financial compensation. At the college and university level, full-time entry-level teaching jobs can pay from $50,000 to $120,000 per year. High school and elementary teachers generally earn salaries ranging from $25,000 to $120,000, with the wide range attributable to varying levels of seniority and teacher educational level. These positions are weekday positions with several months off per year, as well as regular vacations and paid days off throughout the academic year. Pay rates and raises depend on a calculation based on the specific institution, department, and individual qualifications. Adjunct teaching positions, requiring six to fifteen hours of teaching per week, pay from $48 to $110 per hour. As a physician, you may rank lower on the pay scale than others who hold educational degrees, as experience and other factors within the field are formally ranked as more valuable than your nonteaching degree. This may be the case in several nontraditional jobs, especially if you commence a career that is only tangentially related to your medical experience.

Teaching and tutoring for medical licensing examinations can serve as a possible part-time prospect, allowing you the opportunity to work with those aspiring to the medical profession. The pay varies among the private companies that offer such courses but can range from $50 to $120 per hour.

No Rules. See Figure 6.2.

Fund-raising and organizational jobs can be permanent, but most often are temporary. As these positions do not require an MD, the pay and route of entry is

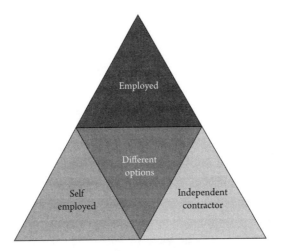

Employed: Hospital administration, Health industry jobs, Regulatory oversight, Scientific research, Medical school administration, Public Health, Government agency jobs

Self-employed: Starting your own business

Independent Contractor: Technical writing, Public education,

Different options: Risk management, Policy, Technology, Laboratory jobs, International health, Regulatory oversight, Disability evaluations, Long-term care

Figure 6.2 Pay structure for alternative work

similar for physicians as nonphysicians. Jacque Jovic, who has worked as a press secretary for a local political campaign, says that payment for this type of job is about $5,000 per month for what is defined as a twenty-hour per week position. However, she explains that the actual demands include twenty-four-hour per day attentiveness and immediate responsiveness to media developments. She explains that the intensity of the work required is generally only sustainable for a few months. The campaigning can be more painstaking with statewide or national campaigns, and the pay for campaign managers and similar positions is higher for more heated races that cover wider geographic regions.

International work, an area of interest for many physicians, can be intimidating with respect to financial survival. Jennifer Furin, MD, PhD, says that a full-time salary for international work is typically $30,000 to 40,000 per year. Dr. Furin says that there is a marked difference between international health clinical service and research. She says that there is generally more funding available for research and that MDs who obtain international research grants are likely to be disappointed if they expect to be able to squeeze in clinical service in addition to research, as the research positions require full-time work. She says that attaining funding for clinical work can be tricky and encourages physicians who are dedicated to full-time international work to be creative in looking for resources and suggests organizations, such as Catholic Relief, Project Blessing, and Partners in

Health, that help place physicians in international clinical projects. In addition, many universities and some nonreligious charities provide limited funding for international health travel or stipends.

Compensation for patient education is much less predictable for physicians. Most physicians who write or give talks for patient education do so on a volunteer basis to promote wellness in their institutions or to increase their professional visibility among patients in their community. Only a few very well-known doctors, typically those who possess a gift for connecting to viewers or readers, receive any compensation for public education. Some of these widely admired physicians include Michael Riozen, MD; Mehmet Oz, MD; Sanjay Gupta, MD; and Drew Pinsky, MD; all of whom the public turn to for medical information, because they communicate easily understandable public health material in a likable, relevant manner. Other physicians, such as Dean Ornish, MD; Andrew Weil, MD; and Caldwell Esselstyn, MD; have written popular health books for the public. Of course, such success stories are few and far between, and unlike the jobs described above, represent a long shot as a career alternative.

Opportunities exist for physicians to write columns in magazines or local newspapers, and compensation varies among the media, but the volume of medical information needed is unlikely to be enough to provide an income. Gail Weiss, an award-winning medical writer, suggests that physicians consider whether writing is going to be a sideline or a career. She says that physician-written articles for nonclinical publications on topics such as medical economics are rarely paid more than a small stipend of about $100 to $150 per article. Public educational writing is more often a complementary endeavor for practicing physicians than a full-time job. More paying jobs are available for physicians as editors or in medical writing companies, and this work typically pays about $50–$150 per hour of work.

It is important to note that many professionals dream of writing. It can be especially difficult for those with great expertise in a specialized field of technical knowledge to ascertain what people are willing to pay for. I would venture to say that those of us with highly specialized knowledge and interests tend to overestimate public interest in our own areas of expertise.

Full-time writing or editing jobs are not easy to find, and the compensation is the same for physicians as for nonphysicians, as an MD is not characteristically a prerequisite. Many doctors at every level offer their public health and technical writing services. This leads to intense competition. It is rare for a physician to maintain a full-time living doing technical medical writing or editing. The pay for full-time work or freelance projects varies from $25 per hour to about $50 per hour. As an alternative, the pay may be per project rather than per hour.

Many doctors have been inclined to write blogs without any financial compensation. Roxanne Sukol, MD, who writes an engaging and popular nutrition blog, says that there are few direct opportunities for reimbursement for such work. She says she runs her blog because she feels a need to continue to write due to the benefits that she sees for her patients. And she says that the time spent in reaching out to the readers of her blog is well worth the effort. With very high web traffic blogs, she says, there can be potential for paid advertising or sponsorship, once a target number of regular hits, in the range of at least forty thousand to fifty thousand per month, is attained. She adds that if a writer in any medium, whether it is magazines or blogs, becomes well known and popular, this can lead to paid speaking engagements and consulting work.

With writing, there is certainly a chicken or egg phenomenon. Practicing physicians often write to promote their clinical services, and physicians in nontraditional careers can benefit by using writing as a means to promote their businesses. Subsequently, MDs who run a reputable company, or are well liked by patients and other doctors, tend to be better received in their efforts to write.

Nonphysician Salaries

Many physicians want to know how much they can expect to earn if they leave medicine. There are a few prevailing rules of thumb. In fields such as the pharmaceutical industry, healthcare organizations, and other companies that employ a large number of doctors, there is an established fee structure for physicians at every level.

In new industries, and in jobs without a well-known precedent, there will be greater variability. It can be challenging to predict a fair salary without knowing the job description, and the profit expectations of the company related to the physician's specific work. In fact, there may be instances when MDs are either overpaid or underpaid depending on individual company profit forecasts.

When a physician works in a company as the only doctor or one of very few doctors in a nonmedical capacity, the customary pay may be determined by the prevalent pay formula for other professionals who provide similar value to the company. Therefore, it can be useful to know what other professionals earn, particularly if you will be involved in negotiating your salary as a physician in a business setting in which you are not playing a physician function.

Data from the US Bureau of Labor Statistics regarding executive salaries shows that executives are among the highest paid workers in the United States. Some top executives of large companies earn from hundreds of thousands of dollars to more than $1 million annually, although salaries vary substantially by type and level of responsibilities and by industry, length of service, and type, size, and location of the firm, organization, or government agency. Median annual wages of wage and salary chief executives in May 2008 were $158,560. Government executives often earn considerably less. While this description is broad, you will, no doubt, be able to gauge where you fall in the spectrum of executives if you obtain an executive position in a hospital, health insurance company, pharmaceutical company, or other large medical service company.

You might find yourself better defined, particularly early in your transition, as a manager, rather than an executive. Managers perform duties such as planning, directing, and coordinating the daily operations of establishments; they also are generally involved in the financial and budgetary aspects of the business. The management occupational group includes CEOs and top-level managers as well as managers of individual functions, such as sales and human resources. Median annual wages of general and operations managers in May 2008 were $91,570. The average hourly earnings of managers in private establishments ($41.86) were greater than those in nonprofit establishments ($34.24) or in local government ($39.75) (USBLS).

If you expect to work primarily among lawyers, you might consider starting your estimate with the background knowledge of attorney compensation. The median annual wages of all wage and salary lawyers were $110,590 (USBLS).

In the political arena, salary data are publicly available, and anyone has access to salary data for elected officials on the Internet or in state or county files. Yearly salaries of governors ranged from a low of $70,000 to a high of $206,500. US Senators and Representatives earn $174,000, the Senate and House majority and minority leaders earned $193,400 (USBLS).

There are an abundant number of salary calculators available on the Internet. They adjust for factors such as region and company size. However, it can be difficult to determine the methods used to obtain data. Monster.com, salary.com, and payscale.com are a few of the sites that have been collecting data for over ten years. The volume may improve the reliability, and it makes the most sense to use results that are consistent with other sources as a gauge. Some potential considerations to look for in your interpretation of salary estimates on Internet sites include bearing in mind whether calculators attempt to report full-time salary, or whether they base calculations on an average of a forty-hour workweek. It may be helpful, if you are negotiating a consulting fee or salary for a job for which there is no clear precedent, to formulate the most similar nonphysician job description and to compare several results using as many sources as possible.

What If I'm Really Thinking about How Much I Will Pay, Not How Much I Will Make?

Other possible endeavors, on the other hand, actually bear a financial cost, rather than offering an income, at least in the short term. Certainly, obtaining further education likely incurs the price of tuition. Workshops and additional degrees can be costly, with markedly wide variability in the range of tuition among different programs. There are ways to help offset the cost, but most physicians who are serious about their supplementary educational goals have told me that they considered the tuition to be worth it. I have not spoken to anyone who regretted paying for an additional degree or certification.

Training courses for billing and coding or other specific medical management at local colleges can run several thousand dollars. Supplemental training courses for complementary medical procedures such as acupuncture or cosmetic injections ordinarily run in the $5,000–$15,000 range for a complete course, most often with a duration of days to weeks. The cost of graduate degree programs, such as MBA programs, which take from two to three years to complete, ranges from $10,000 per year for state-funded programs to $35,000 per year for private tuition.

In rare instances, your clinical or alternative work employer could agree to cover the tuition for your additional training, either partially or fully. It is worth it to check out such possibilities, as you may not be aware of employee packages for supplementary education. Of course, you would likely be obligated to some continued role with the hospital or company, and you will have to weigh the pros and cons of this type of arrangement.

Occasionally, teaching at a university can offer tuition discounts for courses within the university, or at affiliated establishments. This may be a useful method for enhancing your qualifications. However, this may prolong your transition plan, because teaching requires time and preparation, as does taking classes. Some programs offer tuition discounts for teaching assistants, which may require less preparation time than actually teaching a course.

Other resources for obtaining assistance with the finances of additional training include grants, medical societies, and nonprofit agencies. If you have a well-thought-out plan, you could benefit by looking into agencies that support your long-term goals as a possible resource for obtaining assistance with your additional training.

There are loan repayment programs for physicians who want to pursue international medical work or nonprofit work within the United States, and for physicians who follow their calling to become full-time religious clergy. Examples of resources for medical school tuition loan repayment include the National Health Service corps loan repayment program and the clinical research loan repayment program.

Politics is another endeavor that incurs a significant price tag for physicians, rather than a lucrative return. Salaries for elected officials are usually posted publicly on state or county websites, and, as mentioned previously, are generally equal to, or lower than, full-time practicing physician salaries. However, opportunities for speaking engagements, board appointments, and other paid consulting opportunities are generally more available to veterans of the political process than to most physicians.

John Fink, MD, a vascular surgeon in Akron, Ohio, has run for State representative in Ohio. He values the experience, but cautions aspiring physician politicians that politics wants either your time or your money—not your insight or advice, as many well-intentioned doctors may believe. Dr. Fink says that a political party is likely to support a candidate who has a high chance of winning, and who can raise a significant amount of money for his or her own campaign, in the range of at least $100,000–$500,000 for a local campaign. The political party, with more political expertise than the physician candidate, specifies how the money will be spent on their candidate's campaign.

Steve Mehta, MD, a cardiologist in Arizona, was encouraged by his patients to run for office. He agrees that a political campaign is very costly, especially in major metropolitan areas. He says that a physician (or any prospective candidate) would be expected to raise between $500,000 to $3 million to run for a congressional seat and five times that amount to run for senate.

Politics is a field in which there is intense competition. Despite the pressures, time commitment, financial obligations, and likely pay cut involved, being selected by a prominent party as their chosen candidate is very difficult. Physicians are typically drawn to this field as an opportunity to have a positive impact on the community.

Physicians who are interested in writing fiction, nonfiction, or medical information books, often run into difficulty in getting a book proposal accepted by a publisher. Many professionals have turned to self-publishing as a way to publish their material, whether fiction or nonfiction. This can incur the cost of the publishing itself, editing, publicity, and shipping costs. Depending on the length of your book, the cost of publishing may range from $5.00 per book to $12.00 per book, with additional fees for editing, formatting, and other services. It may be worthwhile to consider the costs and expected returns of self-publishing, even prior to initiating a book proposal with a publisher, as a publisher certainly will also look at the anticipated profit. If you, as the author, cannot justify the cost, neither will a publisher.

The Cost of Altruism

Doctors with the objective of devoting their time to nonprofit endeavors vary in their degree of involvement in the financial and managerial aspects of such organizations. For example, many doctors prefer to donate money to nonprofit organizations, while fewer physicians, but nonetheless a significant proportion, like to play an active role in the management of these types of foundations. Therefore, funding issues and budgetary administration are of concern for some MDs, as they follow their dreams of starting another endeavor.

Nonprofit, physician-run projects often incur an economic cost as well. Lee Elmore, executive director of North Coast Health Ministry, a clinic for the uninsured in Cleveland, Ohio, describes North Coast's beginnings, in 1986. An orthopedic surgeon brought up the idea as a way to serve the uninsured. Elmore says that the surgeon demonstrated the community need, suggested a mechanism for stepping in to the gap, and proposed a business model. Initial funds raised by four local churches amounted to sixteen thousand dollars. The clinic began with no paid staff for about two years, and now, has grown significantly as a busy nonprofit clinic, serving patients in Cleveland. Ms. Elmore has helped other people start free clinics over the years as well, and says that the Association of Free Clinics is a very useful resource.

Ms. Elmore explains that there are many resources to obtain funding for nonprofit start-ups and to maintain continued support. In her experience in Cleveland, she used Foundation Center Headquarters and a Library of the Foundation Center, which list organizations that fund projects. There are Foundation Center headquarters and Libraries of the Foundation Center in cities across the country, including New York City, and Atlanta. She recommends actually going to the Foundation Library personally, rather than doing a search online, as the staff in the library can help in narrowing the search for the most relevant funding sources.

In searching for local foundations, it is critical to evaluate whether the foundation missions are in line with your goals as you formulate and write a grant. Guidestar.org is a database for finding nonprofits on the Internet and gives an idea of the budget and size of the individual organization. Some resources for funding include the Robert Wood Johnson Foundation, the Kellogg Foundation, the Annie E. Casey Foundation, the Centers for Medicare and Medicaid Services, and the Kresge Foundation. Many universities maintain resources that can be used by new businesses or nonprofit ventures.

A well-written grant is a good start. Lee Elmore initially learned how to write grants by attending workshops at Cleveland State University. She recommends the book, *Strategic Planning for Dummies*, as an introduction to writing grants and obtaining funding for nonprofit projects. She also recommends the book *Non-Profit Guide for Dummies*, which is particularly helpful with respect to policies when setting up an organization. Ms. Elmore shares that the secret to the success of any nonprofit endeavor lies in building good relationships.

A rheumatologist who has started a foundation to help patients with lupus explains that she has been primarily involved in raising money and then selecting an established organization each year to give the funds to, often designating a specific purpose for the money, such as family support or transportation assistance. She also says that it is important to distinguish the mission of a nonprofit organization, to avoid overlap with other nonprofits, giving a group the ability to do more without competing with other organizations, but instead, collaborating. Several physicians have echoed the advice that it is important in the nonprofit world not to duplicate a service that is already being provided, and that it can be helpful to try to partner or piggyback with an existing entity in order to build a stronger foundation.

Purchit Lacuesta, MD, who has traveled to several countries doing medical missions work, says that she pays for her own travel and accommodations and lives simply while abroad. Some physicians, however, raise funds for their trips, either directly or with the help of service-oriented groups, to help cover the cost of volunteer medical missions, either within the United States, or abroad. Fung Ho Song, MD, who has done extensive medical missions work abroad, including establishing medical clinics in several countries, has raised money for medical equipment and hiring support staff through colleagues that he has worked with, and through churches.

Exit Costs

Planning exit strategies includes allowing for expenses such as medical malpractice tail, outstanding office space and equipment rental agreements, staff salary and retirement contractual obligations, patient record maintenance, collection follow-up costs, and possibly other financial agreements. Many physicians choose to maintain board certification and state licensing even after conclusion of clinical work because some nontraditional jobs require this, and because it leaves the option open for reentry into clinical practice or medical volunteering. This incurs a cost of between $100 to $1,500 per year, and possibly less for physicians near retirement age, because of grandfather clauses in some state licensing policies.

Exit costs are considerably variable, and a blanket number cannot accurately reflect individual cost. Variability depends on factors such as medical specialty, region of the country, population of the town in which a physician practices, and most of all, financial obligations and legal agreements made prior to, and during, establishment of clinical practice.

Overhead costs such as rent of space and equipment can run in the range of thousands to hundreds of thousands of dollars and rarely in the million-dollar range. It is the astute and fortunate doctor who can construct a plan to end a clinical practice well timed with lease agreements. Some physicians continue to rent space or equipment and sublet to leaseholders for additional income or to break even, paying attention to the need to compensate for additional taxes incurred by rental profit. Other physicians prefer to continue to hold on to real estate or medical equipment as an investment and rent or sell when it is advantageous and convenient.

Staff contract end dates may extend beyond the target ending date of clinical practice for some physicians. Additionally, even after the last day of seeing patients, some staff or billing services may be needed for an additional six to eighteen months in order for a doctor to collect payment for patient care. Typically, costs such as advertising are not very expensive for most medical practices and do not present marked expenditure of funds that would interfere with the financial goals of departure from clinical work.

Medical malpractice insurance is one of the most burdensome obstacles to leaving clinical practice. Many medical malpractice contracts are defined as claims made policies. By definition, when a doctor has a "claims made" policy, the medical malpractice insurance company only covers the physician for medical malpractice claims that are filed *while* the physician is covered by that plan. If a physician discontinues the coverage with that company to leave clinical practice, or even to change jobs, the company no longer covers any future claims, even if the incident occurred during the time when the malpractice contract was in effect. The malpractice insurance company typically demands what is called a "tail" payment for any future coverage, which is approximately 2.5 times the cost of a yearly malpractice insurance premium. If this fee is not paid, this could leave an unacceptable, hazardous gap in malpractice insurance coverage, despite the fact that the physician has continuously paid premiums. This system is legal, and it is very common for the high cost of tail coverage to trap physicians in practices that they want to leave. At the current time, there is no real solution for this malpractice insurance system, and the financial implications leave many physicians stuck in a bad work situation, because it is difficult to absorb this particular hefty exit cost. Medical malpractice, in particular, is a limiting factor for many physicians because, unlike office space rental, equipment, and even staff financial obligations, this cost is dramatically elevated at the time of exit from practice and cannot be sold or leased to someone else.

Often, small group practices hire young physicians and provide the bare minimum malpractice coverage in order to lower overhead costs, while maximizing returns for the more senior physicians who already have to deal with decreasing reimbursement rates. However, large healthcare systems are generally self-insured, providing appropriate coverage for their physicians, as malpractice claims affect the whole institution. I have known many young doctors who, unsure of their long-term plans, proactively limited their practice options to large self-insured hospitals, even accepting a lower paying offer, because the cost of future malpractice premiums and future tail coverage is a number that can vary each year, and therefore is nearly impossible to lock in for the future at the time of employment.

Medical malpractice tails are estimated by each individual medical malpractice insurance company, and may change on monthly basis depending on a number of economic factors. Therefore, physicians typically get an estimated quote from the insurance company, and a modification in the actual cost of the malpractice tail may occur several months later when the actual tail is paid. There is great variability depending on medical specialty, malpractice insurance company, and geographic region. A search on the Internet resulted in numerous essays and posts from physicians with stories of malpractice tail surprises, ranging from $40,000 to $300,000. However, I obtained company quotes that generally use a formula of 2.5 times the yearly cost of medical malpractice insurance for tail coverage. At the lowest end of the spectrum, a dermatologist in a small town in a Texas may pay $15,000 per year in malpractice insurance coverage and $30,000 in tail cost. A gynecologist in Cook County, Illinois, would pay about $125,000 yearly in malpractice insurance and approximately $320,000 in malpractice tail fees upon leaving practice.

Conclusion

Approaching the financial aspects of your future goes hand in hand with every other consideration. Knowing some of these facts can help you to narrow down your choices. The numbers are a practical consideration for anyone contemplating a career change. While there will never be hard and fast guarantees, there are guidelines that can help you understand if your professional interest suits your financial needs. See Figure 6.3.

Some doctors feel more comfortable with negotiating than others. Some doctors also feel that they are in more of a position to negotiate than others. Regardless of your circumstances, you might find the above parameters useful as you assess whether your next job offer is equitable.

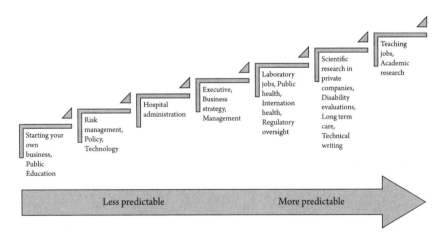

Figure 6.3 How predictable will your salary be?

SECTION THREE

THE ROAD MAP—FINALLY

7

Getting the Right Job

So far, *in theory*, everything sounds great. You recognize that you are not the only doctor who has contemplated leaving clinical medicine. You have clearly evaluated exactly why you want to take your career in a new direction. You examined the features of the professional path that will make you happy, while utilizing your professional and individual talents. You have genuinely assessed your work priorities and read about potential nonclinical options with your own values in mind, in light of important data such as pay, time commitment, job availability, and stability. You have the tools to narrow your search to potential jobs that will work for you. You can finally take the critical steps to go from the hypothetical to the practical and target particular fields so that you can effectively launch your next professional stage.

Some physicians use earlier phases to bridge into new ones, while other doctors construct more planned out, purposeful changes of direction. There are numerous options, and each description of the evolution into a nontraditional medical career is unique, as yours will be. Many doctors, in hindsight, describe for you what they wish they had known. See Figure 7.1.

How Should I Start Looking?

Fortunately, when it comes to finding opportunities, you have many resources at your disposal that can assist you in finding the position that you want. There are three key methods that you can use to open doors to your next career phase. You could find a job on your own by directly approaching employers, you could obtain assistance from a professional, such as a recruiter or a career consultant, or you could start your own corporation. The doctors who have shared their experiences have effectively used a combination of these three key methods, and you will ultimately choose a blend that is a good fit for you and your background.

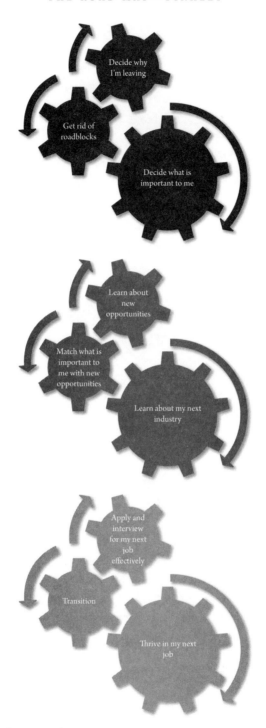

Figure 7.1 Steps to your next career.

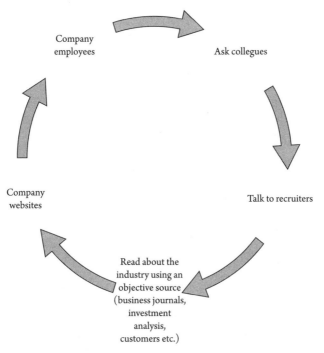

Company
employees

Ask collegues

Company
websites

Talk to recruiters

Read about the
industry using an
objective source
(business journals,
investment
analysis,
customers etc.)

Figure 7.2 Learning about your industry of choice.

Educating Yourself

Now that it is time to take real, meaningful action, you can finally begin to set the stage to implement the job that you want, or start your own venture. See Figure 7.2. At this point, you need to look for a specific position by efficiently using your resources to make your search effective and successful. A broad, all-encompassing quest is likely to be unnecessarily time-consuming and futile. You have much to gain by focusing on one, or just a few, categories of nonclinical career options that appeal to you and satisfy your goals. The reason that you do not need to apply to many jobs in a variety of the different nonclinical areas is that you can get what you specifically want if you first take the time to become knowledgeable and informed about your field of choice. Expenditures of the US healthcare system surpass 2 trillion dollars, with approximately 11%–21% distributed to physician reimbursement for direct patient care. Healthcare is a stable contributor to the economy, providing jobs for a substantial segment of the population. This fact indicates that regardless of the nonpracticing niche that you want to establish yourself in, there is a place for you if you position yourself well.

The first step you need to take in positioning yourself well is educating yourself. Once you focus your job search to specific options, you should broaden your search to many possibilities within those few options. You will reach a more fruitful outcome when you direct your valuable time and energy first to thoroughly learning about the one or two specific areas of nonclinical medicine that interest you, such as management or technical medical writing for example. As you continue to educate yourself about your chosen career direction, you will quickly become considerably well informed about the field, formulating a methodical appreciation of which companies in your exact industry of interest and region of the country are leaders in the field, which are well established, which are innovative, and what they each value. You will develop a keen perception about each individual company's self-defined identity by how they market themselves to clients, to business associates, and to the public.

This initial strategy provides you with the background information needed to present yourself in the best light, highlighting your qualifications and experience in the most advantageous manner. The level of awareness gained serves to help you decide whom you want to contact and communicate with and how to do so, in order to gain the access that you need to attain the type of role that you are looking for. This will appreciably improve your chances of being hired, or of becoming successful if you start your own company. Once you learn about the field, you can successfully create an effective application process. A few simultaneous parallel job searches in unrelated fields such as pharmaceutical product development and teaching can also be useful, but only if you make an educated inquiry into each one, thus it will require more time and energy to do it right. While narrowing your selection and doing your homework may seem an obvious initial step for some, there are too many physicians who get lost looking for alternatives. An uninformed job inquiry is a weak job inquiry. See Table 7.1.

Whom Do You Already Know?

The most common way to find a job is by talking to people you already know. Several doctors in prominent nonclinical positions have looked back and modestly described their career transitions as fortuitous consequences of routine interactions made during clinical work. The method of using your current work environment to platform into your next career would work well for you if you have strong social aptitude and networking skills or have succeeded particularly well in your current position. Using your current work situation to bridge into your next one will suit you if you have demonstrated proficiency in working well on a team. Provided that you fulfill the basic qualifications for the job, your personal skills can provide you with a great advantage if future work associates who have seen or heard about your positive approach in your current setting will be more enthusiastic about working with you. If you have a sensible vision for improving a system in your

Table 7.1 **Pathways into different jobs**

Academic Research	Application through department chairman	Collaboration	Recruiters	Networking
Industry research	Networking	Application through company human resources	Recruiters	
Government Position	Networking	Committees	Application through department chairman	Collaboration
Business	Networking	Application through company human resources	Additional Degree	Collaboration
Insurance	Networking	Application through company human resources	Recruiters	
Hospital Administration	Networking	Committees	Collaboration	Recruiters
Education	Networking	Committees	Application through department chairman	
Public Health	Networking	Committees	Collaboration	
Technology	Additional training	Collaboration	Networking	Recruiters

existing environment, and if you are able to do this without alienating others, you would be well suited to using your current work to transition into your next career, if you would like to get into hospital administration or medical school education, for instance. Staying within the healthcare system that you already work in can provide a simpler job modification, allowing you to maintain part-time clinical work or start a new nonclinical job without having to relocate. You will also be able to bridge what you have already learned about the priorities of the environment that you work in to help you advance in your nonclinical career for years to come.

Many industries described in Chapter 5 lend themselves well to this approach. Medical school education, hospital administration, public health, biotechnology, the pharmaceutical business, and the insurance industry are all areas in which you undoubtedly already know some associates. If you typically maintain positive interactions with others, then you probably have already cultivated a network of colleagues. It will be valuable for you to ask physicians and nonphysicians who are directly or even peripherally involved in that field to share their insights with you about your field of interest. You can share your questions, and gain a great wealth of information from people at all levels within a particular business. You can use this groundwork to gain a strong behind-the-scenes understanding of hospital administrative needs and available posts, for example.

You would position yourself as a strong candidate for administrative or teaching jobs by getting involved in committees and making well-thought-out, beneficial contributions to your organization. The dean of student education at a prominent medical school emphasizes that becoming engaged in medical student or resident education on a committed level can help a physician to catapult into a formal position in medical student education. He observes that many academic administrative positions are homegrown because institutions recognize that they need someone who has earned trust, exhibited leadership skills, and demonstrated empathy. Examples of dedicated roles that can provide you with a real significant experience and differentiate you include serving on admissions committees, taking an active and consistent role in student mentoring, or preparing learning objectives for student or resident education.

On a hospital-wide level, joining risk management or quality control committees are examples of actions that can provide you with experience and visibility to the administrative hierarchy within your hospital as you demonstrate your abilities. This can build a foundation so that you can work your way up in a stepwise fashion to higher, paid administrative roles.

To bridge into the pharmaceutical industry, Dr. Schwartz advises to be interested in what product representatives say and to learn about how the corporation works, the organization, the product goals, and the business goals. He also suggests trying to meet the boss of the reps you know, as well as the boss of the boss. Demonstrating interest resonates well with a company that has needs for MDs. Nonphysician professionals, such as sales representatives and product support specialists are a rich source of unbiased insight and advice into industry. You can learn important details about how the field is organized and obtain direction for useful contacts within specific companies and organizations that you are interested in. This information can eventually help position you to find a job working either as a full-time associate or as an independent consultant for a company that you already interact with in some way.

If you are able to determine how you can fit the needs of a firm, this could lead to your filling an existing opening. For instance, if you discover that a company is dedicated to growth and expansion of quality control, you will be better able to approach your inquiry for a position. Another possibility to consider includes proposing a new position that may not yet exist but that would be beneficial for a business's strategic objectives. You would need to clearly outline how your position would benefit the company, and several of the MDs I spoke with credited this strategy for their success.

You might have innovative goals that do not follow a clearly defined path. If you want to become involved with weight loss and wellness, for example, you could begin by starting a program at your hospital and documenting measurable targets. If you are interested in biotechnology product development, perhaps you can speak with someone at the company that makes medical devices that you already use. Likewise, if you are interested in healthcare guidelines, you may consider discussing this particular interest with someone at the health insurance company that serves your patients, or with the outcomes department of your hospital.

A very important object to keep in mind, however, is that networking does not necessarily mean directly asking for a job. Most likely, your contacts within an organization of interest to you are not in a position to hire new employees. Therefore, rather than alienating your associates by asking them for something they cannot deliver, it is more useful to learn from your colleagues about the industry as a whole, including the work environment, new projects, upcoming company or division goals, who is officially in charge, and who is actually pulling the strings. This can serve to unlock doors for you that you would not have known about otherwise.

Your involvement in your professional association, local organization, or national medical society can lead to useful physician and administrative staff contacts. Your specialty organization can potentially connect you with publishers, health insurance medical directors, and key health policy and public health leaders. Furthermore, your specialty association and similar professional groups are invested in your success as a physician member.

Stepping into the Unknown

A physician who has been a leading clinical research executive at a large biotechnology firm agrees that it can be helpful if you know someone within a large company. In fact sometimes MDs within the nonclinical realm recruit talented doctors from their pool of acquaintances and former colleagues. While this obvious point can be exasperating for doctors who do not have contacts outside of clinical practice, it is certainly not the only way to venture out of clinical practice. You may have a career aspiration that lies completely outside of your current contact sphere. Perhaps you are interested in the biotechnology industry but do not take part in research or interact with medical equipment support representatives nor are involved in your hospital supply committee.

Ashraf Hanna, MD, PhD, vice president of commercial finance at Genentech, says that it does not matter whom you know, but rather what you know, and how strong you are as a candidate. He says that there are many positions for good doctors in the biotechnology field. He states that applications are reviewed even for doctors who do not have experience in the field of biotechnology. Dr. Hanna says that a good way to get to know people in biotechnology companies is to make the effort to participate in clinical trials while still practicing clinical medicine. Because the clinical trials are so important to a company, senior directors from within the companies always get involved, and visit patient trial sites to assure quality. This potential source of interaction can help practicing physicians begin to understand how a prospective employer functions and can help in determining whether the environment would be a good fit. Most importantly, Dr. Hanna explains, biotechnology senior staff looks for strong recommendations when hiring new physicians. Dr. Hanna, who entered the biotechnology field shortly after completing medical school, says that it is an important principal to perform well at your current job, even if you think it might not be right for you in the long term.

Several of your options, such as a biotechnology, healthcare technology, the pharmaceutical industry, insurance review companies, medical communications, or government healthcare agencies, are fields in which there are positions in hundreds of small and large businesses. Each of these companies has individual needs and a different system for hiring. Their company sizes vary, as does their individual expected growth. If you have strong communication and writing skills, and you can highlight your accomplishments and intentions well, you might find that the approach of directly contacting possible employers yourself is the best way for you to make a good impression.

Large businesses often take applications in the human resources section of their websites. It will be worthwhile to devote time and attention to company sites, evaluating whether you really are suited to their business mission. Several recruiters and company human resources specialists explain that most applications are typically filed until openings become available. A follow-up with a phone call and an e-mail to a hiring director or medical director may steer you in the right direction and give you an idea about the company's upcoming needs. It is a good idea to research a company's support materials and website thoroughly so that you can customize your letter of intent and CV to highlight your relevant qualifications, experience, and references. While most MD jobs are not always advertised through human resources, this method will be most effective if used in combination with other approaches. This will allow executives who have the role of acquiring physicians to easily locate your information within the company system once you initiate contact and discuss a possible position, and to confirm that you are serious and dedicated regarding your inquiry.

Richard Smith, MD, MBA, a senior medical director with a leading peer review company, says that he receives many inquiries from physicians who reach him through some form of interaction with the company. He says that while there is a fairly constant need for physicians in review jobs, timing is everything. He explains that he often accumulates many inquiries when he does not have openings, but that he maintains a waiting list, which he refers to whenever the demand for MDs increases. He says that medical director positions may not be in your backyard when you are looking. If you wait, and if you are willing to be patient, however, he says, they likely will pop up in a nearby metropolitan center. The more complete your information is on a company's waiting list, the more likely they are to follow up with you if the information and earlier contacts indicated that you are qualified once a position becomes available.

A useful resource to identify prospective companies within your area of interest is by looking up targeted key search words on the Internet. Useful phrases include detailed job functions such as "medical writing services," "healthcare quality review," "telemedicine," "pharmaceutical utilization," "healthcare marketing," or "healthcare product research" rather than general terms such as "healthcare executive" or "physician administrator." Spend ample time on the links that you find. Specific company website results are far more useful than job title results. Some searches will yield too many minimally related links, or links to irrelevant advertisements. This is the reality of the Internet. There is an abundance of valuable, updated, and fluid information. However, you will also notice a great deal of unedited, unfiltered, inconsistent, and anonymous material.

Healthcare management companies and government healthcare agencies have websites that list openings for positions. Agencies that collaborate with other establishments, such as the Agency for Healthcare Research and Quality, the Centers for Medicare and Medicaid services (CMS), and the National Center for Complementary and Alternative Medicine, often have links to other similar or associated companies. It is valuable to spend time looking up many different companies within your area of interest. Continuing medical education sites are a fertile resource that can help you to identify medically related companies. Because there are so many CME articles posted on a wide range of topics, you can read about the companies that produce devices or provide research regarding medical management, costs, marketing, or a number of possible services based on your own target direction. Industry specific chat rooms and national meetings can be a useful resource for information about prospects, such as the American Medical Writers Association or medical device meetings listed on the Food and Drug Administration website.

Deborah Stein, MD, an internist who primarily worked in student education, says that it can be helpful to contact an individual whom you admire who is already active in your field of interest or a similar field, even if you do not directly know that person. Asking for advice and direction will be useful, and the worst thing that could happen is for the person to simply not get back to you. I have been pleasantly surprised to find that most people who have attained success have been graciously willing to share their advice and experiences for the benefit of other physicians.

While asking for a job can be successful, it is also effective to ask the contacts that you find on company websites for advice on how to break into that specific industry. You can benefit a great deal by connecting with more than one person within an organization. The companies that you will directly contact may or may not have a need for what you have to offer right now. Nevertheless, by speaking with more than one person in the field, you can really gain a well-rounded perspective on your future job. Your conversation with several people at several different companies is likely to trigger your name in future dialogue within that industry.

Several doctors mentioned that small medical companies, especially those owned by MDs, tend to hire physicians through word of mouth. Initiating a collaborative project without placing great emphasis on pay can help you showcase your skills and pave the way for a more official position. Examples of collaborative projects would include writing patient materials for a medical product company on a freelance basis or giving a lecture on your specialty and how it relates to the company's product.

Getting Professional Help with Your Search

Recruiters and headhunters are a useful resource for several reasons. Unlike a company website or a link, recruiters are actual experienced people who will interact with you, listen, and give you a realistic assessment of your likelihood of finding what you are looking for based on your needs and situation. Businesses compensate headhunters to find suitable individuals to fill a needed position. Recruiting professionals expect to speak with you and to offer you advice, guidance, and potential job opportunities, without any payment from you. They also do not have a contract with you, and you have no exclusive formal, informal, or ethical obligation to work with only one recruiter at a time.

April Confessore, a recruiter with Infinite Talent Medical Staffing, says that she receives many calls from physicians inquiring about nonclinical opportunities, and that she generally recommends that the doctors who call her directly contact the HR department of pharmaceutical or insurance companies, or a corporate recruiter, rather than a physician recruiter. She says that she has heard of physician recruiting firms considering branching out into nonclinical placement, but that the physician recruiting industry is already too busy in placing clinical positions, for which there is a high demand.

Most corporate recruiters are very focused and know the details of the professional specialty within which they work with very well. They are experts at describing the work environment, job duties, and expected salaries in the field that they represent. There are specific recruiters specialized in locums work, moonlighting, pharmaceutical jobs, teaching, and other categories. However, recruiters who specialize in pharmaceutical jobs, or technical writing jobs, do not exclusively place MDs, and typically place more nonphysicians in the healthcare field than physicians. They will direct you to potential employers in light of the qualities needed for the job function, more importantly than in light of your background as a physician. Recruiters will give you an idea about the standard experience and background required for the jobs that they place, as well as income expectations. They will not, however, provide you with feedback or assistance in editing your CV or letter of intent or tell you how to present yourself in the best light. Headhunters and recruiters are not there to help you with your transition. They will provide your information to potential employers because their job is to find a person to fit the job—not to find a job for you. It is easy to find a recruiter either through word of mouth or through searching for a recruiter in your specialty of interest on the Internet. Once you make contact with a few recruiters, you will be on their radar when a position for which you are suited becomes available.

Another good resource can be found on networking sites such as LinkedIn, which is currently popular. As you know, prominent leading websites and networking sites change so quickly that within a few months the current leading websites and specific Internet resources listed may already become outdated. Over the past few years, LinkedIn has been a popular and growing site on which one can connect with professional colleagues or alumni from medical school, residency, and so forth. Many health industry recruiters also maintain groups on LinkedIn that one can join or follow without obtaining any type of formal approval, or providing any personal information. These groups send updates with industry information, and frequently post job openings and identify organizations that are a supply of jobs. LinkedIn can serve as a resource of communities that one can join which generate newsletters about business trends in niche areas like health technology or health marketing.

There have been good reviews about following specialized recruiters on the social networking site Twitter. Recruiters and human resources specialists at large companies often use Twitter to post updated job openings. In order to get these postings, you must open a Twitter account and follow a recruiter. To follow someone on Twitter, one must simply decide unilaterally to "follow" a person or organization. An individual or organization that runs the Twitter site does not need to accept or know their followers. This can make the site useful for you if you intend to follow someone who has many updates, but whom you do not plan to interact with, until a position of interest becomes available. There is an advanced search feature on Twitter that can be used to look for more targeted information. One can limit searches by entering information such as location or hashtags, meaning keywords, to expand or focus a search.

Facebook is a well-known and very popular social networking site with a growing number of users. It is becoming common to use Facebook to promote products by creating fan pages of a particular product or business. There are groups and Facebook pages for some professional organizations, and the interactive possibilities are likely to evolve. Branch Out is another new professional connection site. New web services are so fluid that in a very short period of time resources and interactive mechanisms for finding jobs will undoubtedly have improved even more than described here.

You will find that there are a few websites, articles, and courses, devoted to the topic of physicians leaving clinical care. If you are interested, you can also look for medical and nonmedical career coaches specialized in the area of career transitions. There are few medical career coaches for MDs and many career coaches who are not specialized in medicine. A career coach or career consultant is paid by the person who is looking for a job, unlike a recruiter, who is paid by the employer. Career consultants provide services to help you with your resume and your career planning. You may decide to use a coach specialized in professional transitions, physician career development, or overall lifestyle direction. As with recruiters, you can find people either through word of mouth or through the Internet.

Personal and career coaches charge for services such as advice, personal assessment, and CV and letter of intent editing. There are several payment models, such as paying by the hour or paying for a package of services. There is a range of fee structures, and each individual recruiter would have to tell you what they charge on a case-by-case basis. A physician who transitioned into hospital administrative work several years ago, noted that she initially worked with a career coach. She explains that the coach did not find her a job but provided value by helping her feel validated and less guilty about looking for nonclinical work. Another MD says she attended a seminar put on by a nonmedical life coach, which provided her with a much needed nonjudgmental support structure, because she had a lingering hesitancy to take action despite the fact that she was unhappy in her work.

Presenting Yourself

By the time you begin to apply for positions, you will have gained a good understanding of the fundamentals of the business that you wish to work with by reading about the companies in your field of interest and making contacts within the industry. When sending a professional inquiry, it is to your benefit to highlight what you have to offer to serve the needs of the company, in light of what you have learned about the field while doing your preliminary research into your future arena. You can accentuate why you are suited to that field, demonstrating that you are knowledgeable about this industry and not simply looking for an escape from medicine.

It is expected today, more so than in the past, that a CV, letter of intent, and method of approach should be individually directed and tailored to the specific position for which you are interested. Similarly, a brief letter of intent, or a letter of interest, indicating what you have to offer, either in an e-mail or an attachment, is expected to be directed and relevant. Anything less indicates a lack of interest, dedication, and sincerity.

Customizing your CV and letter of intent is not in any way dishonest. Companies and businesses expect you to provide relevant information prominently and to communicate your strengths succinctly. Maintaining honesty and integrity in your job search is paramount to your success. If you decide to send many letters to several universities inquiring about teaching positions, your letter should be addressed to the specific college and department to which you are sending your letter. Additionally, a brief statement relating why you are interested in teaching at that particular university, indicating your knowledge of the institution or department's reputation and strengths, and mission, positions you as a more thoughtful candidate.

A medical director who receives many job inquiries warns not to make the mistake of changing the content of the letter and sending it as an attachment without changing the file name of the attachment. Interestingly, he shares that, because he frequently forwards applicants' e-mails with attached resume and letters to other directors at his company, small oversights often get forwarded to several administrators. He states that nothing screams out "I don't really care and I only have a few minutes to do this," more than sending out an attachment to one company with the file name of another similar company.

This is particularly important for physicians because, sometimes, when looking for alternative work opportunities, doctors may be viewed as arrogant or nonchalant about nonclinical matters. Paul Sweeney, DDS, a dentist who had done extensive medical missions work abroad describes an attitude of "I'm a doctor, show me your patients," or even more striking, "I'm a doctor, I'm here to be in charge," in the area of international health among some American doctors. Physicians educated and trained outside the United States are equally book smart, and often have more experience with physical diagnosis, especially when it comes to diseases endemic to their geographic locations. They often have to deal with an exceedingly high doctor-to-patient ratio and lack of hospital space in crisis situations. Native physicians in countries where American doctors volunteer medical care may lack technology and hands-on experience with newly acquired or donated technology. For that reason, the teamwork approach is ultimately better for patients and physicians alike. Anticipating such details in your next environment (discussed further in Chapter 9) positions a physician to better present him or herself when trying to find an alternative position. Bids for positions of authority should be backed by experience and a balanced attitude.

At the same time, you should approach this process with confidence. As discussed earlier, you have made a rational decision to search for work in a nonclinical field. You can absolutely sabotage yourself if you approach your search for a nontraditional medical job with a sense of uncertainty or hesitation. While some doctors may give a negative impression by acting as if they are loftier than nonclinical situations, others can make the opposite mistake and appear to be embarrassed that they are leaving clinical practice.

Several physician medical directors pointed out that doctors should approach interviews with a sense of direction. Having clear focus demonstrates that you are serious about working and not just looking for an escape. Dr. Schwartz says that motivated statements such as, "I want to make a product that helps with this clinical problem," or "I want to work in marketing strategy," work much better for a physician applicant than vague statements of looking for job.

A good barometer of your likelihood of finding a suitable position is whether your CV and contact letters are sincere and are representative of you, and of what you wish to achieve. As you read the letters to yourself or to someone you trust, you should ask yourself—is it real? If you cringe when you read them, or if you are too uncomfortable to show them to a trusted friend or mentor, this could suggest that you need to make some changes before you send them out.

A common theme that is important for physicians to note is that industry, whether product related or insurance related, is primarily concerned with quantitatively measurable endpoints, in sharp contrast to medical practice. In other words, if you plan to work in a section or division of a large company, your effectiveness will be measured within a specific timeframe and within the goals of your department. It can be difficult for physicians to adjust to this when they have spent years trying to improve long-term overall quality of life for their patients. A cardiologist, while not concerned in detail with the nervous system, takes great care to avoid harming his or her patients neurologically. Yet in business, improving your specific division ratings are of primary importance, often above the goal of improving the health of the company overall. And, often, long-term objectives are not as critical as performance for established deadlines. Therefore, a physician may be misled in attempting to position himself or herself as a strong candidate by stating that his or her goals include lowering overall healthcare costs or improving patient care, when the hiring director's goals are specifically related to lowering cost of *his particular division* relative to other divisions within a large insurance company.

As you begin this job search, it is helpful to remain organized and focused. You may be so busy with clinical practice and all of your other personal responsibilities that you only have time to dedicate to looking for another opportunity intermittently. It is a good idea to keep track of all of your contacts with organizations and individuals either by making folders in your e-mail account or by recording dates and names of contacts. You could also make a point of keeping track of all negative feedback and comments. Use these as valuable learning tools as you continue to better understand your future field. This will help you not only in obtaining a position but also in learning what is important in that field so that you can advance in your next job as time goes on.

Some of the organizations that you will contact may have more pressing issues than hiring a new doctor for nonclinical work. Therefore, it is up to you to initiate professional follow-up. It is reasonable to send an inquiry by phone or e-mail to confirm that your information was received and complete. It is also sensible to ask for a general estimate of when you can expect a response. With rare exceptions, nonclinical work opportunities will not chase you, and it is up to you to promote yourself, and to be persistent in looking for opportunities and pursuing them.

Using Your Strengths

You have a clear understanding of your individual values and abilities, and that has helped you in refining your job options. Similarly, you will more successfully direct your career path when you use your unique strengths to guide you to your optimal method of searching for a job. See Table 7.2.

If you are highly respected at your current work, you will be best served by using your current work contacts to network, as you highlight the well-recognized accomplishments that you have achieved in your own work environment. If you choose to leave your work environment, however, you should remember to emphasize that your colleagues or supervisors are enthusiastic about offering letters or phone calls of recommendation. It is also important to recognize that you may be respected in your current job for any of a number of different reasons, including publications, clinical expertise, innovative approaches, or

Table 7.2 **What are your strongest qualities?**

Peer-reviewed publications
Patient care
Communication Skills
Teamwork
Teaching
Good Speaker
Creative
Focused
Strong exam scores
Strong knowledge base

communication skills. There is more than one definition of performing well, so you do not need to fit the ideal mold of your current job in order to use your current position to platform into your next. One physician I know of was meticulous and always insisted on thorough, comprehensive patient workups. He was not considered to be the "star" of the group because he was often behind schedule and was unable to see as many patients as his colleagues. Furthermore, they often had to "pick up the slack" and see patients who were scheduled to see him in order to keep the pace moving. However, when he left his clinical practice for a medical directorship position, he received high praise because he was very well respected for his conscientious devotion to accuracy.

If you are a talented, articulate, and engaging speaker, you could begin by offering to speak at the organization for which you are interested in working, or for potential clients, if you are starting your own business. At the very least, highlighting your presentations and the feedback that you reviewed in your CV could alert potential organizations of your strong speaking skills, if it is relevant and valuable to your future area of interest.

If you are an articulate writer, or if you are particularly methodical, you could consider contributing articles to a blog or magazine while at the same time highlighting your background and skills, allowing prospective employers or customers an opportunity to get to know you and what you have to offer through your writing. Writing is a positive instrument through which you can use your organizational skills to your advantage. You might decide to write articles that demonstrate your achievements, knowledge, and expertise, and as mentioned above, communicate what you have to offer in a useful and approachable way. Likewise, these activities can help to place you as a search result related to your topic of interest in web searches in the future, which is especially valuable if you are going to be starting your own company. One physician executive I spoke with said that he routinely does a brief Internet search on all potential applicants, and that the information he finds on his own allows for far more useful interviews. So be aware that you have a great advantage in this process in that potential employers and customers will even use information about you that you do not directly provide.

If you are personable, creative, and particularly good at networking, you have to find a way to highlight that strength, potentially through hands-on collaboration with a potential business prospect to display your strengths. This can allow you to cultivate professional relationships, and to meet people who can offer you guidance if your area of interest does not encompass your current circle of contacts. A benefit of this type of interaction is that the experience can help you decide whether the type of career modification that you are considering is suitable for you.

If you are a good communicator, and think well on your feet, personal or phone follow-up can serve to clarify your proposal and allow you to make fluid contacts that could provide you with timely, relevant tips. Personal contact can also allow you the opportunity to relay that you understand the company's needs and expectations, and that you are adaptable. Conversely, if you are not skilled at modifying your message or communicating in person, you would be best served by writing letters of contact, and allowing yourself time to revise and articulate your message carefully.

If you are skilled at business implementation, or if you have strong problem-solving skills, you could highlight your abilities by serving on a hospital committee or in a community-based organization that would give you the opportunity to obtain documentable experience in organizational management. If your qualifications or publications are more impressive than usual, you could benefit from early presentation of your CV and a cover letter that emphasizes your accomplishments. Given that so many resumes and CVs are sent through e-mail, you could easily provide links to your publications and other online supportive material without overwhelming your contacts with numerous pages.

Build Your Experience

If you begin to make relevant connections, and you find that you are not experienced or knowledgeable enough about your field of interest to obtain a paying job, you might conclude that you should build some experience. Given that you are already a highly qualified physician, you can gain the necessary experience and credibility within a reasonable amount of time.

Several areas, including public health, government medical posts, and politics, require years of background and experience before a paying position can be attained. Glenn Graham, MD, PHD, who has worked in the VA system as a neurologist and has a hybrid policy career as well, advises that networking is a necessity and that it is very difficult to move into a government appointed position de novo without prior relevant experience. Jennifer Furin, MD, PhD, also recommends that physicians interested in public health policy obtain practical experience. She explains that a public health administrator or physician in the field in a disaster setting is faced with a scenario in which large numbers of people suddenly need everything from a healthcare standpoint. But, as she points out, it is impossible to give everything at once. Therefore, people who have been in similar situations before are better qualified to prioritize medical needs.

You may choose to volunteer for a professional society or disease-related organization, serve on a board, write relevant articles, give presentations, go to meetings, or take a course or seminar, depending on your situation. As you build your experience, you can maintain contacts and develop new ones in order to better situate yourself to the career to which you aspire.

Jacque Jovic, who is not a physician, has worked as a press secretary for a political campaign and is familiar with the many staffing needs of political campaigns. She advises that volunteering for a political campaign is the best way to start, and that paying positions, such as press secretary, campaign manager, campaign scheduler, speechwriter, and staff coordinator almost always require proven experience and competence, typically showcased in volunteer positions.

John Fink, MD, a vascular surgeon, ran for state representative several years ago. He believes that doctors should have a business background, and some education into the political process as a preparation for a medical career. He says that politics is a tough business. Dr. Fink advises that the way to begin a career in politics as a doctor is by getting involved. He says that if one's goal is to influence policy, the best way to be heard is to raise money. He says that preliminary involvement could include volunteering to campaign for other candidates or raising money. Over time, if the party recognizes that you have the dedication to really effectively work on a campaign, they may begin to see you as a viable candidate who can win. Dr. Fink says that it wasn't until four years after he began participation in local politics that he was fortunate enough to be given the opportunity to run. Interestingly, Dr. Fink notes that his own political campaign was a fascinating experience in many different ways. The entire process was a completely new world consisting of a combination of financial, fund-raising, and political pressures. His experience illustrates the fact that politics is a full-contact sport and involvement is not to be taken lightly.

Running as an Independent is also an option and allows you to maintain control over your political spending, but you do not have the substantial benefits of the financial support, infrastucture, and experience of a well-known party.

Steve Mehta, MD, a cardiologist, was encouraged to run for office by his patients, who felt that he shared their views. He talked to the national congressional committee and was encouraged to run. After losing, he says he learned several lessons about politics that many physicians are not aware of. He says that he had been governor of the American College of Cardiology and had been lobbying on Capitol Hill. But, he says, doctors who want to really understand politics should get involved on a more fundamental level, such as running for state legislature or county chairman.

Dr. Mehta says that his campaign was grueling in terms of time commitment and travel, but that he enjoyed it because of the opportunity to see many parts of Arizona and to meet so many people. He had to modify his practice dramatically; only working structured and scheduled clinical days for about six to eight days per month. He says that, relatively speaking, he started his campaign late, only eight months before the primary, just as the campaign was picking up momentum. He says that had he started a year earlier, he would have had longer to get his message out. Like Dr. Fink, Dr. Mehta says that raising money is a challenge, and that most physicians do not contribute as much financially to the political process as other professionals and professional organizations. Dr. Mehta has plans to continue to combine politics and clinical practice, and plans to use his experience to continue to learn. He encourages physicians to get involved with their professional organizations and to run for public office.

Therefore, if you have to backtrack because your search was unproductive, you could consider networking, volunteering, or becoming engaged in committees and organizations to improve your experience, knowledge base, and visibility.

MBA? Public Health? PhD?

A number of doctors ask whether they should obtain an MBA as a way to attain qualifications for a nonclinical career. This is indeed a debatable question, as many physicians obtain MBA, PhD, or public health degrees even without the intention of leaving patient care. There are different degree paths to public health jobs as well, including MBA (masters of business administration), MPH (masters of public health), or PhD (doctorate of philosophy). Questions frequently arise regarding whether an additional degree will be redundant and superfluous, or whether it will serve to help distinguish an MD from fellow MDs looking for alternatives to clinical practice.

Barbara Shapiro, MD, MBA, an obstetrician, has a healthcare MBA, which she pursued because she wanted to position herself for a medical directorship of her OB/GYN group. After she completed her MBA degree, however, she felt that she learned much more than she had envisioned, including how to make a business plan and marketing plan and how to look for measurable objectives in medicine or in business. She brings up the point that she could have learned some of the basics of business management, including understanding income statements and balance sheets, by reading finance books on her own during the weekends. But, she explains, she gained a great deal from working on assigned group projects during her MBA courses, which required group interaction and a combination of skills learned in several different courses and were subject to practical feedback from her professors.

Dr. Shapiro started her own business in physician advertising and patient education and she says that not only did her MBA open doors for her and provide her with credibility but also it taught her how to evaluate the value of her business strategy in her new company. She states that as a physician thinking about business there may be critical factors that are overlooked simply due to a lack of knowledge. She says of her new view of medicine after she completed her MBA, "The eyes do not see what the mind does not know." This example illustrates how the actual knowledge gained from an additional degree such as an MBA or MPH can help a physician to further understand the nonclinical issues at hand. The knowledge gained can serve to satisfy the physician making the career transition even more than the degree can serve to impress a future employer, as a physician typically approaches such a program with a self-motivated learning objective.

Richard Smith, MD, MBA, says that he had already been a medical director at Blue Cross Blue Shield for seven years prior to obtaining his MBA. He explains that he wanted to understand business better, and that, just as an MD teaches a doctor the language of medicine, an MBA teaches the language of business. He explains that the end product of an MBA combined with an MD is a mold of the two elements. One can better make the equation of medicine and business balance if one understands both sides of the equation.

He explains that in the field of healthcare management, including utilization review, an MBA is not particularly important in entry-level jobs, where clinical judgment is critical. He says that he looks for physician candidates with experience, which he acknowledges can be hard to get when you do not have any. He says that in the esoteric area of utilization review, a doctor should have extensive experience in the trenches of clinical medicine and have attained good clinical judgment and perspective on the appropriate use of diagnostic testing.

This requires a strong medical knowledge and an up-to-date ability to form a differential diagnosis. However, in higher-level positions, such as senior medical director or chief medical officer, an MBA is preferred, but in his opinion might as well be required, due to the balance of the interplay between the business matters and medical concerns.

An MD supplemented with an MBA, MPH, or PhD typically does not in itself lead to job offers or recruitment. However, it allows a physician the opportunity to learn and to demonstrate interest on a committed level, analogous to the strategy of volunteering or serving on committees and boards. In contrast, however, demonstrating dedication by serving in a local capacity can often offer results that are limited to your current setting, while a formal degree is much more recognizable among a wider community.

Expect the Unexpected

As you steer your way toward achieving your dreams, it is important to remain patient. Many doctors have reiterated that there are nontraditional positions for MDs, but that they are not generally advertised. There is also a wide range of types of jobs, some easier to attain than others. However, be prepared for unanticipated opportunities and contacts. Dr. Brian Duncan shared an observation with me that I found particularly insightful, "The harder you work, the luckier you get." His statement accurately describes most of the doctors' experiences who told me that they were lucky, but also had put in time and effort laying the foundations for their nontraditional jobs. *The key for many is that the process of laying the groundwork earlier was enjoyable for them,* and that is why they describe their opportunities as lucky.

There are common principals in approaching all of the alternative avenues, such as patience, persistence, and doing your homework in the field. Once you research the individual type of industry and then the specific companies within that arena, you will easily discern the detailed subtleties in the most suitable approach for each individual industry and company. Generally, the pharmaceutical industry, insurance industry, biotechnology industry, hospital administration, and student education, are the most well established nonclinical routes with clear precedent. See Figure 7.3. However, even in the more unique directions physicians have succeeded and attained great satisfaction.

Jennifer Furin, MD, PhD, of the Brigham and Women's Hospital Department of Internal Medicine and the Department of Global Health Equity, developed a global health residency at Harvard because she saw that formal training in the many facets of global health would be beneficial for doctors who want to effectively do international medical work. But Dr. Furin herself says that she

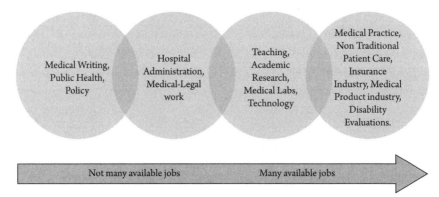

Figure 7.3 Are there many available jobs?

broke into the field of international health indirectly, photocopying articles for Paul Farmer, MD, and Jim Kim, MD, while she was a medical student. She says that they were involved in a very small organization at the time, allowing them to get to know her. She says this gave her the opportunity to go to Peru when there was an outbreak of multidrug-resistant TB. Dr. Furin made a consistent effort to continue in international clinical work throughout her medical school and residency years. After years of experience, adapting to the contradictions in healthcare, such as the scarcity of simple x-ray equipment overseas, contrasted with extensive diagnostic workups in the United States, Dr. Furin started a parallel residency-training program at Harvard Medical School, with a focus on a preparation in international health and care of the underserved. She

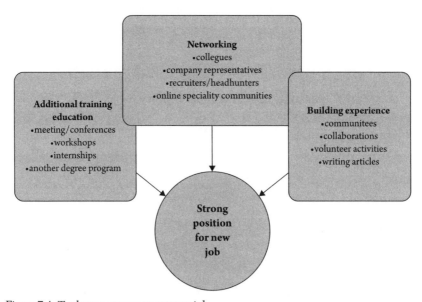

Figure 7.4 Tools you can use to get new job

felt, after her experience, that physicians would serve their patients better if they gained a clear understanding of the demands of international medicine, including prioritizing crisis care, unexpected procedures, limited resources, and introducing new medications and treatments into an established medical setting. Dr. Furin emphasizes that doctors interested in a new field should not consider any job beneath them because they believe that they are overqualified. She stresses that exposure and working in the field you are interested in at any level can be a resourceful route of entry.

Surprisingly, as you examine just a few potential fields of interest comprehensively, rather than casually evaluating numerous job scenarios, you will uncover useful tips and make worthwhile contacts. As you deepen your involvement and widen your circle of contacts, you will become aware of more opportunities in your area of interest and you may even stumble on the best fit for you. You will learn both from your directed search as well as from inadvertent connections along the way. If you have dedicated your time to thorough research about your future field, you will be well equipped to evaluate all opportunities and to obtain the inside scoop on whether a given company or position is right for you. Opportunities often emerge when you aren't specifically looking for them, but they tend not to become apparent if you aren't looking at all. See Figure 7.4.

8

The Physician Entrepreneur

Starting one's own business is something that many doctors aspire to but, for understandable reasons, are hesitant about. Physicians are intricately involved with the shortcomings of the medical system as well as the enduring need for improved treatment options for medical conditions. This serves as a catalyst for some doctors to probe for methods to improve medical care and healthcare delivery. The idea of starting one's own business can be attractive to entrepreneurial physicians who want to proactively address unmet problems in healthcare and be their own boss. If you want to become a physician entrepreneur you must possess a great deal of self-confidence and a personality that can tolerate risk. You must also have a life situation that can withstand the prospect of delayed achievement of your goals and possibly a large financial investment. Innovative ventures and new projects can provide stimulating opportunities for doctors. As finding nonclinical jobs does not follow widely established instructions, starting one's own business, either in the medical field or completely outside of medicine, can seem even more like an expedition in the wilderness. See Table 8.1.

If you choose to start your own company, your business plan should be well thought out and functional, as well as innovative. Instead of researching nonclinical fields for employment opportunities, you will instead devote your initial research to learning about how to run your own company and studying the potential market, pricing, and promotion for your product or service. It will be helpful to seek information regarding the progression of similar companies and experiences of other entrepreneurs as you graph your strategy.

Starting a Business

If you decide to start your own medical or nonmedical business, this requires a greater investment of your time and attention than working for an established company. Your enterprise may be healthcare website, a clinic to serve patients with specific health problems, a healthcare investing company, your own medical-device

Table 8.1 **The similarities and differences between starting your own business and finding a job**

Nonclinical Job	Starting Your own Business
Learn about the goals of the company that you work for	Learn about the product that you will provide
Can find a job on your own or can use a recruiter	Can market your business on your own or can hire a marketing service
Negotiate salary, bonuses, benefits	Negotiate costs of overhead and price of product
You will have a job description	You will create your own job description and job descriptions for everyone you hire
You must please your boss	You must please your customers
You must do your job well	You must make sure everyone in your company does the job well—*or you will have to do it yourself*
You can get a promotion	You can expand your business
You can get laid off	You can go bankrupt
You can continue to succeed and learn from your achievements and your mistakes	You can continue to succeed and learn from your achievements and your mistakes

company, an imaging facility, a coding and billing company, a weight-loss clinic, a stress management enterprise, a parenting organization, a wellness institute or magazine, a physical therapy facility, a new way to deliver healthcare or streamline the process of healthcare, or any healthcare product, patient service, or physician support. Any of the examples above and numerous others could be a way to use your medical background to build a business that preserves what you value about medicine. Many doctors have gone out on their own to start companies. Given that each new business endeavor is unique, there is less of a recipe with respect to any aspect of the transition—whether it be finances, lifestyle, business growth pattern, or business duration. Nevertheless some basic principals apply to all types of business.

Fill a Gap

You need to first thoroughly research the demand for your product or service. This step is generally the easiest for physician business owners because, as most

have told me, they started their businesses as a response to a deficiency in medical services, either for patients, other physicians, or the healthcare industry itself.
See Figure 8.1.

Cheryl Miller, MD, a physical medicine and rehabilitation specialist in the
Southeast, started an ancillary medicine staffing company with her physical
medicine and rehabilitation group to fill a gap for community physicians.

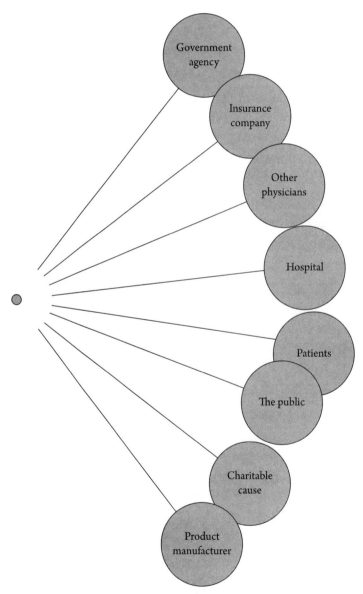

Figure 8.1 Who needs or wants your service or product?

Who is willing to pay for your service or product? *It may not be the same answer as whoever **needs** it.*

For years, she and her physician partners provided high quality rehabilitative medicine and therapy for patients and also became efficient at billing and collecting. They insisted on the highest standards of billing and a thorough understanding of the business side of their practice, including regulations.

They formed their medical staffing company in response to community physician groups who had rehabilitative therapy needs beyond the capacity that Dr. Miller's group could accommodate in their office. In addition, some of the physician groups expressed that they were struggling financially. Dr. Miller's group practice responded to these two problems by forming a company to provide ancillary services to neighboring groups at the physician client's offices, overseeing scheduling, billing, and collections, while collecting a management fee.

She says that she and her physician business partners had to work hard to learn how to juggle payroll, taxes, credentialing, and employee laws, as well as employee management and quality control. She explains that initially there was an astronomical learning curve because medical business is very regulated, and that compliance and following policies is of utmost importance. Her value to physician clients, in addition to providing a needed clinical service, was in mastering the understanding of policies, therefore allowing clients the comfort of avoiding managing what they viewed as the intimidating process of running a business. Many successful business owners have followed the same general principle of expertly mastering tasks that are overwhelming to others.

Dr. Miller adds that marketing a medical business is very challenging, but that her company had built-in advantages because they already knew physicians who needed their services. However, she cautions that getting your foot in the door in a medical office in order to acquire new clients is challenging and certainly not for everybody. She says that the difficulty of the task of acting as a product representative for her own business services when she attempted to expand her business was an eye opener. Additionally, Dr. Miller shares that as Medicare and insurance payments change somewhat unpredictably for ancillary services, the profit margins can unexpectedly diminish, and that can make it difficult to survive as a small medical business. If one has to deal with lower profits, a decision has to be made regarding the pursuit of increased volume weighed with the additional time involved.

Filling a gap is essential. Knowing how to manage a task that others find overwhelming can also give you an edge. And adjusting to changes in income and regulations can be an ongoing issue for a business in the health industry at any point in time.

Focus on Quality

Most importantly, it is essential that you provide a good quality product that you are proud of. Demand for your product alone will not keep business flowing. You will be responsible for properly assessing pricing for your product, examining the competition, and distinguishing your product or service in a meaningful way. You must examine how the production and delivery of your service can be done in a profitable fashion and how to manage every aspect of your company. For the long term, you have to remain focused, as you will need to follow through with support and trouble-shooting with respect to your product.

Renu Virmani, MD, president and medical director of CVPath Institute, providing consultative and research pathologic services to government and private businesses, is a pathologist who has had a self-described "weird career" path. She trained in cardiovascular pathology and then worked at Vanderbilt, and for much of her career worked as a pathologist for the armed forces. She later started her own nonprofit company, CVPath Institute, doing preclinical work for medical devices and pharmaceutical products. Her company works with thirty to forty firms at a time, doing pathology evaluation and testing as well as evaluating results from other labs. She also gets clearance from the FDA for companies and laboratories.

Dr. Virmani says that she thinks entrepreneurial doctors can make a difference in products that come on the market, and can help maintain high quality in these products. Her staff of approximately forty-five people includes five MDs, two PhDs and several masters' level scientists. Yet, Dr. Virmani emphasizes that she started small, with minimal investment. She initially rented space and purchased some equipment to put her lab together. She says that she expanded her company slowly, buying more equipment and hiring more staff as business went well. She credits her success and steady growth to the fact that she maintains high standards. She says that due to her insistence on quality, her customers have been satisfied with her company's services. This has allowed her business to grow by word of mouth, which she says is more effective than expensive advertising.

Dr. Virmani advises doctors to maintain a manageable investment, control costs to avoid debt, insist on providing excellence, and always remain familiar with the regulations involved. This story illustrates a critical principal that many successful physician entrepreneurs have followed. It is important to start any new enterprise at a volume at which you can maintain at high quality. Growth and expansion can follow if that is your goal, but preservation of consistent standards established early on is a key to the longevity of a new company.

A Business Plan

You must have a realistic business plan and an understanding of the costs of running your business. Starting a business can require a great financial investment and risk, and client growth may be slow. Evaluating the market, pricing, and maintaining product support and development are daunting tasks. You may decide to start a business in which you receive compensation from government or nonprofit agencies, from for-profit companies, or from individuals. Physicians who run their own non-patient-care businesses say that constructing a plan prior to starting a business is critical. There are unexpected costs to consider in starting a business, such as insurance and legal protection for your business; equipment; office space; salaries, benefits, and training for your staff; advertising fees; and compliance and licensing costs.

Barbara Shapiro, MD, MBA, a gynecologist, explains that she secured a clinical position with a prominent single specialty group after completing her residency. She explains that she was very busy clinically and experienced a pleasant camaraderie and fair treatment among her colleagues. However, she noted that while her group was growing and excelling clinically, there was a general lack of understanding of the business side of medicine among her partners. She says that insufficient follow-up with regard to billing had not been a significant problem prior to her joining the group in 2001. As reimbursement rates declined, unpaid bills from insurance companies began to have a more serious effect on the balance statement of the practice. With the support of her partners, she obtained an MBA at a well-respected university while continuing her clinical practice at a reduced level, aiming to lobby for a medical directorship position.

She returned to her practice and initially took over the marketing for the group. She built a website for the practice and also began doing content writing and website graphics for patient education. Her proficiency in marketing and web design allowed her to expand to other physician group clients, and eventually she left her clinical practice completely. While her marketing business had been an unplanned consequence of her MBA degree, she feels that her studies provided her with the tools to start her own business. For example, she states that what she learned in her healthcare MBA program taught her how to do a market analysis for her business, construct a business model with measurable goals, design a sustainable business plan, effectively market her services, understand state regulations, and direct her own company's need for a lawyer or an accountant for targeted tasks. She says that initially, while she had very little overhead, her revenue was low because she had not yet built a reputation that would allow her to charge a competitive fee for her work. She advises that a physician who wants to start a company devise a business plan that is workable and one that can provide an income despite the hidden costs of running a business. She also emphasizes that, as a doctor, she is better able to grasp her customers' objectives and to gain their confidence as she advises them on marketing strategy, echoing several physicians who have stated that even when providing a service that may not traditionally be delivered by MDs, a medical background and experience as a physician can make other doctors more trusting and receptive.

Undoubtedly, if you start your own enterprise, as opposed to looking for a job, you will face the challenge and achieve the rewards of being responsible for the financial health of your new enterprise. A solid, healthy, and realistic business plan is the fundamental cornerstone of your project.

Work Hard

Most physician business owners felt that their high quality orientation and efficient management skills helped to give them a better net income than they had been attaining while practicing clinical medicine. But this often came at a significant cost: time. They generally concurred that the responsibilities associated with running a business allowed them little or no time to practice clinical medicine themselves, even if their business provided clinical services by employed MDs.

A group of physicians who have succeeded at their own laboratory based medical businesses explain that they worked as hard as, or harder than, they had as practicing physicians. They emphasized that they know everything about the business and that often they find themselves doing work that they hired others to do, because they are meticulous about detail and timeliness. This inevitable aspect of taking complete responsibility for a company can lead to a particularly demanding work schedule with little work/life balance or boundaries.

One way that some physicians protect against the burnout associated with running a company is by partnering with co-owners. You might choose to form a business with partners or by yourself. If you decide to work with partners, your company might gain some advantages, but you must fulfill the basic requirement that you work well with each other in order to benefit from your individual strengths and to manage your differences productively.

Anthony Valenti, MD, cofounder and co-owner of a busy telemedicine company says that starting a business is immensely time-consuming. He says that his initial motivation was that he wanted to create a business based on how he and his partners wanted to work, not how a corporate supervisor told him to work. His most important objective was achieving the freedom to practice medicine in a way that prioritized quality over quantity. He explains that several doctors who initially worked together to start this company dwindled down to a few because of the time commitment and financial risk involved in starting the business. He admits that he works hard, often putting in 100–110 hours per week, typically working weekends with few days off per year.

He explains that in running a medical business, one has to make a choice between growth and quality. He says that in his company, the hiring process is extremely stringent, and that he only hires physicians who have been recommended by someone personally known to him or one of his business partners. While this maintains physician quality, it limits growth and therefore limits the availability of his company's services. Additionally, he says that he limits the number of patients that physicians can evaluate per hour, and insists on person-to-person contact with the referring MDs. He has a strong understanding of medical errors and feels that his company, because physicians run it, minimizes errors. He admits that this decreases revenue while increasing work.

He also insists that such quality-driven practices and patient-based decisions would not be allowed in non-physician-owned businesses, as he has been encouraged by nonphysician associates to increase the numbers of diagnostic tests read per hour, as this would translate into higher profit. He and his co-owner—also a physician—refuse to make such changes, insisting on high quality because they understand the nonquantitatively measurable value to patient outcome.

He advises medical business owners to seriously evaluate the balance between what produces revenue and what is revenue consuming. He says that as a physician entrepreneur, he had to decide what he valued. For instance, managers decrease owners' workloads and improve workflow for the whole company by double-checking schedules and taking care of paperwork, clients, and so forth, but do not directly produce revenue, and therefore their salaries decrease net income.

He says that he has made decisions that were not the best business decisions, in favor of good medicine. He thinks that physician-owned and managed models for healthcare delivery will likely become more pervasive in medicine as more physicians are feeling the contradiction between what they should do for patients and what they are asked to do by employers. Dr. Valenti emphasizes that running a business is hard work and that there is a marked sacrifice to family life. But he is proud of what he built and of the trust he has gained from his clients over the years.

It has become clear to me, from speaking with Dr. Valenti and several of the other physicians I interviewed, that being a physician entrepreneur takes a great deal of time. Often there are trade-offs between time, profit, quality, and volume. See Figure 8.2. You may decide that a highly qualified, well-compensated staff can save you time and improve quality, even without improving profit. As part

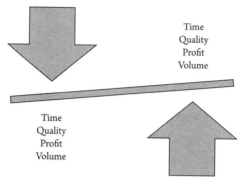

Figure 8.2 Weighing the trade-offs in running your business.

of the business plan, these factors will need to be proactively addressed in order to prevent burnout and to share responsibility for some tasks associated with your project. I also have learned, from many of the physicians I spoke with, that the time and effort involved in making these drastic transitions result in achievements that they view with great satisfaction in the long term.

Master the Rules

Physician entrepreneurs also have to be experts when it comes to understanding regulations and often must adapt to evolving rules. If you decide to participate in running a medical lab or similar type of facility, you should indisputably know the regulations regarding accreditation and billing for professional services and interpretation. Conflicts of interest policies are often subject to frequent modification, so it is best to maintain a strong, updated grasp of these regulations. Be proactive in learning state and federal regulations. Use resources, such as your state medical board and specialty board or society, to fully understand the regulations involving your work or the work of those you will agree to supervise. You are far too educated to rely on casual conversation with administrators or other physicians as a resource for your knowledge about policies.

Amanda Singh, MD, is an anesthesiologist who had been in practice with her husband. She, like several other doctors mentioned, noted uncollected bills and a lack of follow-up by their billing department for their medical services. But she was too busy clinically to follow up on billing matters herself. In addition, when she discussed the subject of medical billing with her fellow anesthesiology associates, they did not fully grasp the complex and changing codes and rules. She made time to take billing and coding courses and began by taking over her own professional billing follow-up, but not her husband's. When she discovered that she was doing a better job than her husband's billing service, she took over her husband's billing as well. A few years later, confident that she was proficient with complicated coding, she expanded her billing services to a few MD friends, charging a percentage of collections, and then expanded her billing company even more from there. She found that her detail-oriented persistence was effective.

She found that she enjoyed the work, was good at it, and decided that she wanted to run her own billing and coding company. Now with eight employees, she explains that she had to leave the practice of anesthesiology due to the responsibilities of running her business, that she is as busy as she was when she worked as a clinical physician, and earns a comparable income, but has a more flexible work schedule. She says that marketing was never a concern for her, but she thinks that marketing can be a substantial part of the job for physicians who need to expand in order to maintain a volume necessary for a suitable income. Her biggest lesson learned is that she has to be very hands-on with overseeing her company and that, while it does get easier with experience, her own meticulous hands-on management style is the reason for her success. She emphasizes that her own control of details is crucial and warns physicians that starting your own company does not lead to semiretirement. She firmly believes that if she "lets go" in any way the quality of her business will decline. She works hard in order to maintain the efficient income for herself and her clients and to continue to offer high quality for the longevity of her company.

Dr. Singh echoes the concept that a physician should understand all aspects of running one's own company, even if others are paid to do the task. Oversight and a continued visible presence are necessities.

Get Help If You Need It

Dr. Frank Dachtler, director of marketing for Healthsource Chiropractic and Progressive Rehab gives insight into a franchise chiropractic business, which offers a few different models of medical business ownership, allowing for more of a business formula for doctors who want to start their own business but crave some structure in the process. Unlike starting a business from scratch, these models of business ownership provide assistance, and a method for an entrepreneur.

Dr. Dachtler, a chiropractor in Ohio had been a busy clinician with several chiropractic offices of his own. After attending a presentation given by a management group, he joined what was then a small franchise concept in chiropractic care. Dr. Dachtler liked the philosophy of a chiropractic franchise because it created unity and decreased competition among area chiropractors. The company, Healthsource Chiropractic and Progressive Rehab, expanded dramatically in the years after Dr. Dachtler opened the second franchise. Now Healthsource Chiropractic has 320 clinics in 43 states and is continuing to grow. Dr. Dachtler stopped seeing patients as a chiropractor as he transitioned into the role of overseeing regional developers, who in turn oversee individual franchise owners. He explains that Healthsource Chiropractic has been named the fastest growing healthcare franchise and has been featured in *Franchise Times* and *Entrepreneurial Magazine*. After having practiced and running offices himself, Dr. Dachtler has been pleased with the opportunity to raise the bar in chiropractic care.

Dr. Dachtler explains that an investor can become a regional manager by purchasing a geographic region to develop a Healthsource franchise for $250,000 to $1,000,000. The investor who owns that region then takes the responsibility of regional marketing to attract chiropractic office franchises in the region. This regional manager/entrepreneur then collects half of the franchise fee from chiropractic offices in the region that join Healthsource and half of the management fee (7%) of gross profits, while guiding the chiropractic clinics in their business. Dr. Dachtler explains that some regional developers manage forty to fifty clinics, while some manage one or two. Additionally, franchise owners, in contrast to regional managers, invest a $29,000 franchise fee to set up an individual Healthsource franchise, and then manage the office, with the methods provided by Healthsource. Dr. Dachtler says that franchise owners and regional developers typically work forty to fifty hours per week.

There are opportunities for doctors to branch out into business using management guidance and sharing profits. Depending on your skills and interest—whether it be equipment sales, real estate development, or healthcare management—you can find a hybrid of running your own business while partnering with a larger firm.

Finances and Details

As you formulate your business plan, you must evaluate whether your project demands a financial investment and whether you will take that responsibility yourself or attempt to obtain funding from investors. In the early stages of a business start-up, there is likely to be a net income loss rather than a gain. Thus most physician business owners that I have spoken to maintained a backup plan at the beginning.

Many doctors have a great plan for a service that is acutely needed in areas such as patient education or patient care quality improvement. But the medical system is not always structured to pay for some of the services that are of value to society. Therefore, exploring ways to be compensated for important work that may not fit into the current healthcare payment structure, either by obtaining funding through grants, providing value to an established company in health product manufacture or insurance, providing a direct service that the public is willing to pay for, or serving a government agency, is part of the challenge that many doctors have had. Physicians who have productively redirected their professional work to an entrepreneurial endeavor have effectively succeeded in this task. Dr. Katrina Firlik, cofounder of HealthPrize Technologies, highlighted in Chapter 3, describes her company as providing direct health improvements to patients (her goal as a physician) and corresponding financial value to pharmaceutical companies, who ultimately profit from and pay for the service.

Several physicians, in starting their own businesses, say that they have been concerned about timely payment for nonclinical services. For this reason, some have used billing services or attorneys to help protect against delinquent payers.

You will also need to make a decision about a marketing strategy and whether you would like to manage this aspect of your company as well or whether you will hire a professional marketing firm. Most businesses benefit by having an online presence and, as with other aspects of running a business, the creation and maintenance of a website may be outsourced, for a cost, or performed by physician business partners, saving short-term cost in money but costing time.

Outside of Medicine

If you are interested in starting a business in a field completely unrelated to medicine, you may have a disadvantage in lacking experience and actual knowledge of the behind-the-scenes workings of your new field. Some doctors, in approaching the restaurant business, for instance, would do best to begin by running a franchise instead of starting from scratch with a completely new idea. Franchises such as food service establishments, preschools, or fitness and recreation businesses, require a predetermined initial investment and a degree of direction and regulation. This can offer a blend of entrepreneurship and support that doctors may find useful if they want to completely step out of healthcare.

If you already know what you want to do, and you are currently charting out your transition, you need to evaluate your future line of business by connecting with people in that field, particularly if your new arena is unrelated to medicine. For example, if you dream of starting your own fitness center, restaurant, or tutoring center, you will need to look into business models of franchises versus individual enterprises to get you started in understanding your nonmedical industry of choice. You must evaluate the initial financial investment and learn how to run that particular type of business. While you are already a step ahead of those who still need to decide what to do next, you need to provide yourself with the background that will be crucial to your success. You may choose to formally pursue training with classes, internships, and certification. Or you might instead depend on reading and talking to others who have already done what you want to do.

Making Lemons into Lemonade

Starting a new enterprise can be an exciting way to venture out of medicine and use your unique talents. Taking responsibility for every aspect of your venture can be both thrilling and frightening. Some describe a feeling of being "exposed," as every aspect of a company's image and success or failure reflects on the owner. But it can indeed be satisfying to effectively "fix" even a small aspect of a broken system. Certainly improvements in public health and preventative care can have a dramatic impact on people's health in ways that are not currently compensated adequately. Medical errors and poor outcomes are not given basic manpower in the current healthcare structure, but instead are most often dealt with by penalties after the fact, which is marginally beneficial for patients at best. Given the complexities of the healthcare system, it is up to doctors to find ways for these and other important functions to take priority and to be properly reimbursed.

9

Accepting the Job: Before and After

Making the Switch

There are many options for the transition process of starting "something else," with regard to both your job combination and your timetable. It is important for you to decide whether you ideally, as well as practically, want to devote your time to your new endeavor exclusively or in combination with clinical work. You could consider phasing in a new career while you phase out of your current one, for a short-term mixture. You might want to continue the hybrid combination of medical practice with your other interest for the long term. You may, instead, choose to definitively conclude your current job completely once you find a new one. See Figure 9.1.

It can be useful to remain somewhat clinically active, but it can be difficult to balance a clinical position with a nonclinical one. Joseph McClain, MD, an

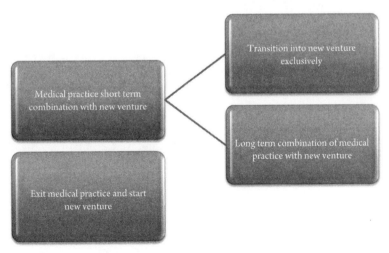

Figure 9.1 Transition paths.

oncologist, started working part-time in the field of utilization review almost twenty years ago, when it was still a fairly new arena. Because he was both unable to find full-time work in the utilization field and because he was unsure of the longevity of his ancillary position, he remained clinically active for eight years until the field expanded and he became a vice president of operations. Similarly, you might experience a gradual or speedy transition and you might want to be certain that you like your new undertaking before leaving your clinical job. Nevertheless, regardless or your personal comfort level with transition and your new direction, you will not find yourself unable to find a dependable job if things do not immediately work out according to plan.

Fast or Slow?

How soon do you want or need to find a new job? How patient are you? If you are starting something new because you have to leave medicine, or you are so frustrated with medicine that you cannot or do not want to be a clinical physician anymore, then you probably want a faster timetable. The urgency involved in such a situation may make the rate at which you could begin to obtain income from your next job more important to you than satisfaction of other professional aspirations. If you still love medicine and your day-to-day work, but you want to pursue something else, you may decide that you would be happier with a measured transition that ensures an enjoyable encore to your current job.

In the short term, the combination that you choose depends fundamentally on practical factors. These factors include your anticipated income from the two fields, tangible progress in your new endeavor, and your professional risk tolerance in making this change. In contrast, the long-term combination that you will eventually become comfortable with depends on the factors considered in Chapter 4 that you have already spent a good deal of time contemplating. These include your degree of interest and dedication to medicine, as well as your intensity of interest and dedication to your new field.

Your available time will certainly play a critical role in the balance of the many factors at play. Can your schedule realistically handle a new career endeavor in combination with your medical career? Or do you have an abundance of time to dedicate to both medicine and a new pursuit in the short term? How about in the long term? How many hours per day or per week do you picture yourself working in medicine or in your new field? Are you planning on a fusion of two endeavors and expecting financial compensation from both or only one of them? You will undoubtedly note that your current practice overhead will not take a break, even if you want to. As noted in Chapter 1, decreasing clinical work by 50%, for example, may not translate into directly decreasing your income by 50%, but possibly by much more, depending on your overhead.

The late Harold Klawans, MD, combined his career as a renowned neurologist with his career as an author of nonfiction and fiction books. His novel *Chekov's Lie* describes the challenges of balancing the two absorbing professions. He explores his own unforeseen sense of being pulled in many directions as a neurologist and a novelist. While he does not tidily weave a pretty conclusion to the dilemma, it is interesting reading for a physician considering entering into a new arena.

Another important factor to keep in mind is how long you want to remain in your new field. Is it just a professional detour or a long-term plan? If you have always wanted to write a textbook, or to design a new physical fitness method, you may be ready to get back to medicine after that goal is completed. Similarly, if you want to temporarily leave medical practice to raise your young children full-time for a few years, you will want to leave the door open for reentry into medicine at a later time. In contrast, if you are financially and personally ready to retire, you may be interested in a nonclinical pursuit that will easily wind down into full retirement in a few years.

Your own perceived level of professional uncertainty has a significant impact on whether you feel comfortable leaving medicine, and whether you think that you may eventually choose to return to medicine again in the future. Most physicians who change direction do not return to clinical practice as a full-time source of employment but rather continue to progress and advance in their new fields for the long term.

If It Sounds Too Good to Be True....

Enthusiasm, perseverance, and confidence are all helpful on the road to building your success in a fresh, alternative field, but only when they are combined with a good heaping of careful, well-thought-out, caution. As discussed in previous chapters, you are not alone in contemplating a career outside of clinical medicine. And, unfortunately, because of the widely known phenomenon of recent physician dissatisfaction, there are assorted traps out there, lurking and waiting for the stereotypical burned-out doctor. The physician who wants, and possibly even needs, to continue to earn an equivalent income while avoiding the pressure, time commitment, and litigation concerns of clinical medicine, can, regrettably, be easy prey.

Stories of doctors who have made costly professional errors demonstrate that it is wise to proceed with caution in order to avoid making a serious mistake that could result in even greater stress than that annoying denial of payment. It is essential to take the high road and only accept opportunities that will not tarnish the durable professional reputation that you, thus far, have worked so hard to maintain. Several doctors I spoke with emphasized that it is especially critical at a transitional stage to protect your assets and to avoid accepting any arrangements or contracts without your eyes wide open.

Many of the stories that I have been told share several common themes and lessons. One is to beware of physicians or administrators who sound naïve. This situation will eventually prove to be troublesome for you in one way or another. Either you are potentially dealing with someone who is dishonest or with a careless businessman whose negligence can cause you to have trouble down the road. The best advice is to wait for a better opportunity and to insist on transparency in all agreements. You should only accept a position that sounds exactly the same as it looks in a contract. Anyone who tells you-"we don't normally use contracts" absolutely should not normally be doing business with you either. And, as one doctor I spoke with told me, you may find yourself reading about that person in the local paper in a few years. Stay away.

Beware of Pitfalls

Nontraditional jobs, like clinical jobs, are almost all authentic. But there are some things that you should watch out for. Any job in which you are hired as an MD to supervise and sign off on a large number of ancillary medical professionals should be questioned. You could be unwittingly accepting a position that thrives on dubious billing practices, of which you may be unaware. Become familiar with billing and coding laws regarding your time spent with patients. Signing off and billing for a professional doctor visit for patients who were not seen by you but by a clinical extender whom you "trust" or who "is really good" can land you in hot water very soon. Do not take responsibility for other professionals' work or bill for anything out of the ordinary. It is well known that there is a dire need for regular physicians to do regular patient care, and you should never rush to accept an unorthodox position, even if the assured pay is much higher than in traditional medical practice.

Another error that can snag physicians looking for part-time work is the "pill mill." In this setting, physicians are hired to manage large volumes of patients requesting narcotic prescription refills. Again, such a corrupt setting is rare, and there has been an increase in safety measures to counteract and clamp down on this type of setting, the state of Florida being a particularly positive example. But you should be wary. A physician with whom I spoke warns of this type of job. He admits that he was not in a position of clout when he was searching for part-time work, while recovering from a serious injury himself. He left the dubious position when he discovered the true expectations of the job, and he paid more money in medical malpractice tail costs than he had actually earned by working. He also cautions, "not knowing the rules is never an excuse."

Hazy Lines

Online medical sites that provide people with medical advice and information are relatively new when it comes to matters of liability. Dr. Sukol says that employers view bloggers as a new concept bringing up new issues that people have not had to deal with before. Judy Fine-Edelstein, MD, who has written content for a health-related website advises to clarify issues related to malpractice coverage and medical license regulations. The issue of who provides coverage of malpractice liability for MDs has been unclear for doctors, many of whom describe medical blogs and informational medical writing by physicians for the public to be new territory for medical malpractice insurers and healthcare institutions alike. Additionally, websites and magazines that typically employ non-physicians may be less prepared for issues related to physician liability. Readers may also have unrealistic expectations, as the "MD" after your name may prompt many to jump to the conclusion that you must be in charge, and therefore held to a higher level of responsibility than other contributors and writers on the same site. It is helpful to proactively address questions about physician availability and patient questions and to define who is legally responsible for readers' interpretations of content.

It is important to understand where the line is drawn regarding responsibility and compensation when you are a physician employed by an institution. For example, who is responsible for liability coverage if you are a doctor working at a hospital and you write an advice blog on your own? Additionally, who collects the fees if you are doing medical malpractice work when you are identified as an expert based on your work at a prestigious hospital? Your employer might be legally entitled to collect compensation, especially if it is your employer who is covering your overhead and expenses.

Dealing with changes in regulations and grey areas can offer new, stimulating excitement for some and unacceptable uncertainty for others. Whether you view yourself as a pioneer or you prefer to stay in well-established terrain, spelling out the policies is a vital prerequisite to your success in alternative medical fields. In situations where there are no clear parameters or precedents, you can initiate the discussion and insist on clarifying the issue. While it may seem tempting to let vague issues slide, particularly if you are concerned that your new idea is tenuous, you have much to gain in the long run by establishing yourself as a credible forerunner in your innovative field.

Disappearing Acts

In some cases, physicians have all the right groundwork in place, including great ideas, a workable business plan, and even a team approach for a novel, forward-thinking project. However, for many reasons, innovative ideas can fall short on funding. Dr. Fine-Edelstein says that one of the pitfalls of pursuing an alternative career path is sensibly preparing for an original project and watching prospective funding fall through. This can happen for many valid reasons, including the fact that funding a new project may just fall lower on the list of priorities for a healthcare system or hospital than well-established services. Tenuous funding or support does not invalidate your project or plan but simply requires a greater level of preparation. Stories of successful projects that were at some point halted or delayed because of loss of funding or restructuring of departments are common. When setbacks such as these are dealt with the right way, they can eventually be used to lead to future opportunities.

Therefore, it is important to take the necessary steps to apply for funding for new projects and first-time positions, keeping in mind that things may not work as planned. If you maintain a backup plan to continue income-producing work and continue diligently investigating other funding alternatives, your patience and responsiveness to constructive criticism will most likely pay off. Many success stories include rejected grant proposals, delays, and setbacks. Persistent preparation and ingenuity in the face of bumps along the road are necessary, especially when your plan includes new ideas or projects.

Emerging fields can offer new, exciting opportunities. They can, however, also prove to be short-lived. A physician who trained in hypnosis in the 1970s recalls an environment of promise regarding this therapeutic technique. Among some physicians, hypnosis was hailed as the cure-all for a vast array of patient health problems, including substance abuse, obesity, depression, anxiety, and high blood pressure. Training courses proliferated, and doctors felt that they could simultaneously help patients noninvasively and attain a new income source. As time went on, the treatment became less fashionable for physicians, patients, and for payers alike.

On the other hand, other concepts that have flourished, such as thrombolytic therapy for cerebrovascular disease, epilepsy surgery, or electronic medical records, were initially viewed with skepticism. It is worthwhile to maintain a tempered and balanced attitude toward novel concepts, as it can be impossible to predict the success or failure of budding medical developments.

Did I Say That?

Several MDs have also told me of the experience of being misquoted in the media. This can affect doctors in clinical practice as well as in nontraditional fields. Physicians who are involved in alternative professional activities are sometimes unprepared for interviews and other media interaction. This can cause doctors who are sincere and unguarded to be misquoted.

A number of physicians have looked back at their own interviews or transcripts and were distressed to see, for example, that they seemed to be over-representing their qualifications or relayed an inaccurate appearance of conflict of interest. The vast majority of media representations of doctors' work and projects are genuine. Good communication and follow-up, and even requests of transcripts prior to publication, are typically well received and helpful for doctors and the media, who have a strong interest in presenting accurate information.

Contracts

It is critical to review contracts in detail. It sounds too obvious—but too many people do not follow the general principal of completely understanding and agreeing with everything that they sign. Many physicians choose to hire an attorney to review contracts. But it is not enough for you to hire an attorney who understands your contract in detail. An attorney who frequently works with MDs advises, "A lawyer is not an agent or an employment negotiator. A lawyer's job is to review a contract to make sure that the agreement is legal—not to make sure that it is fair, or that it matches verbal agreements," (unless you specifically ask your lawyer to clarify confusing sections to make sure that they match verbal agreements). You should not sign a contract with confusing sections at all. Attorneys often point out confusing legal jargon, and one attorney explained to me that one of the common ways that he protects his clients is by pointing out verbose confusing clauses that essentially say "everything in this contract can be cancelled by us, but not by you." You are smart enough to read and understand a contract. If the wording is unclear or does not match your verbal agreement, return it unsigned and request clear language. And then make sure that you agree with the terms of the contract completely. It is up to you, not your attorney, to decide if the arrangement is fair.

More often, an attorney's role is to advise you in the case of a dispute regarding a discrepancy between the terms of the contract and an actual action taken, either by you or the person with whom you share the contract. Hopefully, this will not happen. But, you will serve yourself well if you invest the time and money necessary to ensure that a contract contains the terms that you want *in the first place*. A physician who says he wasted time and money in a lawsuit with a former colleague advises, "Don't hurry into something that could backfire financially or professionally because you are feeling rushed to make money, manipulated by prospective employers, or even accused of being 'difficult' by future partners." An honest business partner or employer will quickly and efficiently clear up language in a contract to match verbal agreements.

If you have agreed to a work condition without a written agreement, you will experience much more difficulty if you have a disagreement down the road about the terms of your employment, termination, or compensation. A good rule of thumb is to avoid casual partnership agreements.

A major key to avoiding pitfalls is confidence. There are numerous well-paying reputable options for you in clinical practice and in nonclinical fields, regardless of your circumstances. Your persistence, patience, adaptability, and honesty in looking for a satisfying career change will most definitely pay off. Feeling rushed or reluctant, in any way, on the path to alternative medical opportunities can open the door to poor decision-making on a doctor's part. Do not waste your time with compromises, and do not allow anyone to take advantage of you. Another important principle is to avoid accommodating temporarily unfair or unacceptable circumstances in the hope that you will revisit controversial issues at a later time, when you feel more secure.

Be completely cognizant of the financial risks and business plans of future partners with whom you may become entangled. As with any partnership, the terms may vary, and partners may even justifiably decide to agree on unequal investments, responsibility, or compensation. But you have to decide, along with your partners, on conditions that are satisfying to you.

A New Environment

Many physicians with whom I spoke emphasized that the environment is different in the nonclinical sphere. As there is no formal route of entry into nontraditional medical work, there is no residency and thus no preview for physicians who wish to transition into nonclinical careers.

There is significant variation in staff support and other resources within every type of research setting. Lewis B. Schwartz, MD, describes the environment at Abbot Laboratories as supportive. He says that in the pharmaceutical business there is leeway for doctors to move around in different roles within the industry. He explains that medicine is just one of many functions in industry in contrast to traditional clinical practice, where medicine is the highest function. He informs physicians that they will have to answer to nondoctors and that, for some, this can be an adjustment. He says that he has continued to value the opportunity to learn from nonphysicians, as his nonphysician colleagues are smart in a way that is different from the way that physicians are smart. For example, in designing business strategy, Dr. Schwartz shares a principal that he learned that is quite different from how physicians think. This principal is, "A strategy is not a strategy if the opposite is ridiculous." In other words, trying to improve client satisfaction is not a strategy, because the opposite—trying to *decrease* client satisfaction—is ridiculous. However, trying to improve a product in a very specific way, or making a new product, is a real strategy that can be tested in a tangible way.

Lisa Manning, DO, a cardiologist who only worked for a few years in clinical practice after completing her residency, similarly describes the pharmaceutical industry as energetic and innovative. This is in contrast to what most physicians have expressed to me about medical practice, where the setting is conservative and possibly guarded with the exception of a few cutting-edge institutions.

Richard Smith, MD, MBA, learned that a physician has to understand the language of business and be able to look at the big picture. A physician who typically treats one stage of a disease but not other stages may not initially appreciate establishing treatment guidelines that are consistent and uniform but that focus less on that physician's area of expertise.

Many physicians who complain that they are not fairly compensated simultaneously complain that "other doctors" are. It has become commonplace for physician specialist associations to lobby for fairer payment models by allowing themselves to become divided from other physician specialties, competing rather than working collaboratively. For example, cognitive physicians who do office-based work object to payment models of procedural specialists, while procedural specialists criticize what they perceive as lack of real value provided by nonprocedural doctors. This attitude of division and competition between doctors is not well received in industry and reflects poorly on doctors who continue to express such grumbles.

Ashraf Hanna, MD, PhD, currently vice president of commercial finance at Genentech, has worked with several companies in the biotechnology industry and describes the environment as encouraging and innovative. He observes that the standard among peers is to motivate people not to order or intimidate people. He says that senior level clinical physicians coming into the biotechnology field may have to adjust, as directive behavior, which may be tolerated when coming from prominent, highly productive physicians in clinical medicine, is not effective in industry leadership.

A notable difference between clinical practice and other types of work in the corporate setting, academic teaching, and public health fields is that physicians and nonphysicians in nonclinical positions are subject to evaluation in the form of scheduled regular reviews and constructive feedback. Numerous nonpracticing doctors have hailed the nonclinical environment as markedly less defensive than medical practice. There is a strong insistence on right and wrong in the medical setting. For instance, when a physician receives an average or below average review on a patient satisfaction survey, the administrative response is either one of the two extremes of "what will we do about this problem doctor?" or "the patient is crazy." Most physicians agree that moderation and constructive improvement is far too rare in the clinical setting.

Most industry jobs are full-time jobs. But some positions are more receptive to part-time work. Glenn Graham, MD, PhD, has worked in the VA system in an administrative capacity and describes work at the VA as having the advantage of the infrastructure to provide salary support for a physician who wants to combine clinical work with administrative public health duties. In his experience, the VA is a place where physicians can innovate in healthcare and play a bigger role in guiding healthcare delivery. Similarly, academic posts often allow for a combination of clinical work and administrative duties within the same institution.

Corporate environments, like the medical environment, evolve with time. However, a difference is that when a company grows or changes, providing new services, new subdivisions are formed to perform the added task. In the healthcare setting, new tasks, such as filling out additional checklists and forms, are often performed by existing doctors and nurses rather than by new employees. In the corporate setting, new jobs and duties are generally compensated by new titles and corresponding pay raises as a job description *formally* expands to include additional duties. Similarly, nonclinical corporate physicians who perform their duties well obtain promotions, with increasing responsibility and pay, an uncommon occurrence in clinical practice.

Business-related duties, such as bargaining and getting a good deal are not the primary job for a physician in clinical practice, but may be a side job. In nonclinical work the business aspects are far more likely to be the whole job, with a side note to avoid harming patient care.

Jennifer Furin, MD, PhD, describes international medical work as a very different environment as well. She says that there is so much to learn but that good-hearted American doctors can make the mistake of thinking that they can tell experienced doctors in other countries what to do. She says that it takes time to get acclimated to the setting, often with significantly less availability of blood tests, x-rays, and other medical facilities. For many reasons, including the change in environment, Dr. Furin recommends going to international medical service trips with well-established groups, at least in the beginning.

Fung Ho Song, MD, who has done medical missions work, often serving Korean populations in Russia, Mexico, and North Korea, has been particularly aware of, and sensitive to, laws regarding restrictions on religious practice in countries such as North Korea. Similarly, physicians who have traveled with Christian church–sponsored medical missions in China, for example, have been particularly careful to respect laws regarding religious practices or evangelization, even when the funding and support for the medical assistance is provided by a religious organization.

Your Transition into a New Environment

Admittedly, the feedback that I have received regarding job satisfaction in the nonclinical setting has been markedly more positive than the feedback from physicians who continue to practice clinical medicine. It may be worthwhile to keep in mind that the higher reported levels of professional satisfaction may be in part due to the fact that most of these nonpracticing physicians are in their second or third jobs and therefore have attained the maturity of age and experience as they approach their work and adapt to their environment. Undoubtedly, in making a career change, you will take a dive into a new environment without the benefit of formal "preview" internships. You will never be required to train as much as you did to become a doctor. But you can use the experiences gained in your training and work as a physician to arm you with the qualities needed to succeed in your next career chapter.

Gaining an appreciation for your new environment will help you find a new position and more importantly, find satisfaction and success in your new position.

10

You Will Always Be a Doctor

Once you ultimately make your transition into the career of your choice, I hope that you will feel a genuine sense of satisfaction. I wish you the best as you experience the gratification of building your new career and begin to enjoy the success that you have worked so hard to attain.

And you will always be a doctor in some way or another. Whether you have decided to remain in the medical field, as a hospital or healthcare management administrator, as a student educator, or as a biotechnological device designer, your background in medicine, working with people, will serve you and others well. Your personal patient experiences and medical knowledge will always keep you focused on the true big picture not just the corporate bottom line. Your conscience in making decisions will be guided not only by theoretical ideas of access to care but also by real experiences of the difference that timely access to good care makes.

Additionally, you have the benefit of knowing the deep importance of the doctor patient relationship. You know how external factors can interfere with patient perceptions of their doctor's judgment. You know that informed patients, with doctors who have time to listen to subtle details and to thoughtfully answer questions, have better short-term and long-term outcomes. You have also had experience with the shortcomings of the medical system and have wished that your job as a physician could be unhindered by unnecessary obstruction and helped by better tools. You know that you have chosen your nonclinical career as a way to enrich your work and your life and that enhancement of the healthcare system is a possible by-product of your career change. Physicians don't enjoy the hassle associated with health care delivery. But doctors also realize that the stress associated with bureaucracy and lack of transparency in the health care system is compounded for patients, who must bear the angst of a medical illness along with the uncertainty of whether medical bills and ambiguous coverage will also result in serious financial problems. We all realize that the anxiety associated with working as a doctor is limited compared to the fact that all of us will one day share the experience of being a patient or having someone who we care about become a patient.

There will undoubtedly continue to be opportunities to use the skills learned in medical school, residency, and beyond in your next endeavor, even if you decide to leave healthcare altogether. Father David Milad, DO, a Christian Coptic Orthodox priest, was a practicing internal medicine physician when he left medicine to follow his calling to the priesthood. He says that clergy are in the minority of doctors who leave clinical medicine. He has known physicians who left because they did not like medicine and have chosen completely different paths, such as starting a retail business. Father David, however, loved medicine but felt a strong pull toward a different calling. After he became a priest, he observed marked similarities between medicine and spiritual care, more so than he had anticipated. Father David says that the interviewing skills and the methodical systems for addressing problems that he learned as a physician are tremendously helpful to him when giving advice and helping people as a priest. He even says that his approach to follow-up with individuals in his congregation often reflects the diligence in follow-up that he practiced as a physician.

Father David says that the reaction to his decision from his physician colleagues at work was very supportive. He specifically entered into the priesthood to care for youth and he says that his physician colleagues saw the need for clergy focused on young adults, even when they were from a different religious background.

Often, retired physicians choose to take on completely new projects and apply much of what they learned in medicine. Fung Ho Song, MD, a retired radiologist, had worked with medical missions during his years of clinical practice. Now, as a retired physician, he has set up medical clinics in Korea and Russia. He raises money through churches and hospitals to buy medication and equipment and ships these supplies overseas. He has hired Chinese physicians in North Korea to staff a clinic and he arranges for physicians from the United States to train them. Interestingly, he noticed that the patients at one of his outpatient clinic locations did not have enough to eat. Given that the lack of such a basic need can interfere with effective medical outcomes, he responded to the problem by establishing a low-cost bakery nearby to provide adequate food to the patients. Often, in a second career, unobstructed by institutional billing quotas, a physician has the freedom to tackle harmonizing activities at the same time.

When undertaking completely different interests, years of medical experience with patients can color and shape a physician's next career chapter. An East Coast anesthesiologist who was specialized in neurosurgical procedures involving epilepsy surgery and intracranial monitoring moved from a big city to a smaller town when her husband received a new job opportunity. Financially stable, she decided to pursue her dream of painting. She had spent her medical career monitoring patients in the semisleeping state for the rare types of neuro-surgery that required patient alertness rather than complete unconsciousness. After her years of interacting with patients as they made subliminal semicon-scious comments and observations, she focused on painting with shapes and colors that gave people comfort and contributed to a state of relaxation. Soon she she began receiving requests to paint murals in people's homes and some restaurants instead of framed paintings, as she had expected. Often, in making a transition to a completely nonhealthcare field, physicians can use the privilege of observations made through years interacting with people in unique ways.

Another physician, a psychiatrist, had had a long-lasting hobby of basketball. Understanding children's needs for discipline and constructive feedback, he began a basketball instructional organization in order to teach children a skill that could give them confidence, but also to model child interaction techniques for parents. The method of demonstrating for parents how to gently coach children was something that he had been lacking the resources to do in clinical practice.

Many physicians who choose to work less or not at all contribute to the world around them by using tools obtained from their years as physicians. A nonprac-ticing physician who left practice when her children were young tells me that she started a Facebook group for adolescent teen girls to discuss social issues with some adult moderation. She had no model for this type of role or community and found a positive response. She serves as more of an advisor than a mom to the girls and is able to understand that adolescents often want the guidance of a trusted adult who is not as involved in their day-to-day life, very much like the role of a doctor.

A retired physician started a group aimed at helping local immigrants with assimilation, providing guidance and basic necessities. With their understand-ing of the complications of obtaining healthcare, they help people apply for health insurance and medication coverage. Because of the importance of par-ents' understanding a new educational system for their children, the team guides parents to ask the right questions and help their children to get the most out of their education.

Oliver Sacks, MD, the best-selling author, is an inspiring example of the type of blend between science, humanity, experience, and empathy that can speak to people in a unique way regardless of their level of education or age. Dr. Sack's articulate and touching portrayal of neurological illness in the novel *Awakenings* inspired a movie of the same name.

Looking Forward

You can continue to find opportunities, either in your community or in other communities or even in other countries, to continue to care for patients with the time commitment of your choice. Many nonpracticing doctors feel a desire to give time to programs teaching about health issues, such as parenting, nutrition, caring for the disabled, or other subjects that they may have found lacking while practicing. Your own personal and close-up insight into public health knowledge and the impact of insufficient health awareness on patients, their families, and their communities, can help you to respond to the needs with the right approach to reach the public.

You have many opportunities to use your medical knowledge and experience, even if you choose a completely nonclinical career path. If you choose to open a restaurant of your own, you can be a better employer because of your experience with health disabilities and work-related stress. Even if you were fed up with disability forms for patients who seemed to be malingering while you were practicing clinical medicine, you can create a work environment that does not contribute to such behavior. If you become involved in the media, you know from experience that children, adolescents, and adults respond differently to information and influences from the media and that it has a significant impact on their lives.

As with any job search, there are so many subtleties. A medical director, a hiring executive, or your new customers may be more focused on criteria that encompass tangible characteristics when they are looking for a physician to fill a nonclinical role. Your opportunities in being hired increase as you fulfill these tangible characteristics. Your chances for long-term success in your next job, however, improve dramatically if you also fulfill the important nontangible criteria, even if no one else can clearly define those criteria during the initial hiring process. This includes creativity, reliability, patience, flexibility, honesty, and integrity. Any function that you have will impact people in some way. After having seen patients in their times of stress and uncertainty, I hope that you will always view others through the lens of compassion as you pursue your next career chapter.

INDEX

page numbers in italics indicate illustrations